Philosophy and Medicine

Volume 150

The Philosophy and Medicine series is dedicated to publishing monographs and collections of essays that contribute importantly to scholarship in bioethics and the philosophy of medicine. The series addresses the full scope of issues in bioethics and philosophy of medicine, from euthanasia to justice and solidarity in health care, and from the concept of disease to the phenomenology of illness. The Philosophy and Medicine series places the scholarship of bioethics within studies of basic problems in the epistemology, ethics, and metaphysics of medicine. The series seeks to publish the best of philosophical work from around the world and from all philosophical traditions directed to health care and the biomedical sciences. Since its appearance in 1975, the series has created an intellectual and scholarly focal point that frames the field of the philosophy of medicine and bioethics. From its inception, the series has recognized the breadth of philosophical concerns made salient by the biomedical sciences and the health care professions. With over one hundred and twenty five volumes in print, no other series offers as substantial and significant a resource for philosophical scholarship regarding issues raised by medicine and the biomedical sciences.

Lisa M. Rasmussen • Søren Holm
Editors

50 Years of Philosophy and Medicine

Springer

Editors
Lisa M. Rasmussen
Department of Philosophy
University of North Carolina at Charlotte
Charlotte, NC, USA

Søren Holm
School of Law
University of Manchester
Manchester, UK

ISSN 0376-7418 ISSN 2215-0080 (electronic)
Philosophy and Medicine
ISBN 978-3-031-95174-9 ISBN 978-3-031-95175-6 (eBook)
https://doi.org/10.1007/978-3-031-95175-6

This Springer imprint is published by the registered company Springer Nature Switzerland AG
The registered company address is: Gewerbestrasse 11, 6330 Cham, Switzerland

Foreword

This book, number 150 in a series of 150 books, celebrates the 50th anniversary of the Philosophy and Medicine series. The series founders, H. Tristram Engelhardt Jr. (1941–2018) and Stuart F. Spicker (1937–2013), inaugurated the series by coediting the proceedings of a *Symposium on Philosophy and Medicine*, *Evaluation and Explanation in the Biomedical Sciences* held in 1974 in Galveston, Texas, to "take the philosopher beyond problems and issues which today are subsumed under the rubric 'medical ethics.'" The new form of medical ethics that Engelhardt and Spicker were referring to had emerged 5 years earlier, in 1969, when philosopher Daniel Callahan partnered with his next-door neighbor, psychiatrist Willard Gaylin, to form the Institute of Society, Ethics, and the Life Sciences, which is now known as "The Hastings Center." This center originally focused on ethical issues at the two ends of life: human genetics (e.g., eugenics, gene editing), population control (abortion, birth control, sterilization), and death and dying (withdrawing life support, euthanasia; now called medical aid in dying (MAID)). In that same year, 1969, medical school faculty founded the Society for Health and Human Values (SHHV) to encourage concern for human values in the scientific and practical education of healthcare professionals. The SHHV would become a progenitor of the American Society for Bioethics and Humanities (founded in 1998). Two years later, in 1971, André Hellegers founded the Joseph and Rose Kennedy Center for the Study of Human Reproduction and Bioethics, now known as the Kennedy Institute of Ethics, to create a scholarly basis for the emerging field of biomedical ethics by publishing a bibliography and an encyclopedia.

In 1974, the publications of these emerging institutions were officially christened "bioethics," by the Library of Congress, which declared that this would be the name under which they would be catalogued. But as Engelhardt and Spicker surveyed the scholarly landscape in that seminal year, 1974, they realized that a core scholarly discipline, philosophy, was absent from the mélange of names, institutions, and objectives newly baptized, "bioethics." So, they held an interdisciplinary *Symposium on Philosophy and Medicine* in Galveston and published the papers presented at the conference as the inaugural volume of the Philosophy and Medicine series.

I made the acquaintance of both editors at a 1974 summer Institute on Medicine and Morals, which purpose was to inform and entice philosophers and lawyers to reflect on ethical, legal, and philosophical aspects of medicine and biomedical sciences. Engelhardt was then, and would forever remain, a boot-wearing Texian libertarian philosopher-physician questing after moral foundations, who, not unlike Socrates, liked to prod people out of their comfort zones. Stuart was, and would always be, an affable east-coast philosopher who, with a twinkle in his eye, used gentle humor, anecdotes, and historical references to make learned and humorous comments that informed his audiences and put them at ease.

As it happened, some colleagues and I co-edited a clinical volume for the Philosophy and Medicine series that would test Engelhardt and Spicker's mettle as editors. That book, *Legislating Medical Ethics* (volume 48), published a series of papers and documents on a 1986 New York State law mandating written evidence of a patient's or surrogate's consent as a prerequisite to writing do not resuscitate (DNR) orders. New York's Commissioner of Health claimed that the state's DNR law would ensure "respect for the autonomy of the patient; ... protect a professional staff from the humiliation of unethical charades ... [and] reduce ... unjustified and sometimes cruel decisions to subject patients to useless cardiopulmonary resuscitation (CPR)."

Physicians call these so-called unethical charades "show" or "slow codes," practices they believed were necessary to protect patients against "unjustified and sometimes cruel" CPR. One study presented at the conference found that the New York law neither eliminated nor diminished show or slow coding. The lawyer directing the ethics commission that drafted and proposed the DNR law tried to suppress this "bad press," demanding that Engelhardt and Spicker expunge that study from the volume. Facing the threat of lawsuits, the co-founders steadfastly refused to delete that study or to abandon the volume; instead, they insisted that printing the paper would implement a scholarly practice of airing both sides of a controversy. The published book included the controversial study.

The current editors of the Philosophy of Medicine, Søren Holm and Lisa Rasmussen, embrace the founders' commitment to scholarly integrity and support the founders' mission of publishing works at the interface of philosophy and medicine, such as the *Handbook of Analytic Philosophy of Medicine* (vol. 119, second edition, 2015) and *The Fragility of the Philosophy of Medicine* (vol. 147, 2023). Yet, following the founders' precedents, they have expanded the scope of the series to include such subjects as *Islam and Bioethics* (vol. 146, 2022). Then, now, and in the future, the Philosophy of Medicine volumes have been, and will continue to be, an indispensable resource embracing and supporting the full range of scholarly endeavors in biomedical ethics that, in the words of the series' founders, "explicate medicine's philosophical presuppositions."

Robert Baker

Emeritus Professor
Department of Philosophy
Union College
Schenectady, NY, USA

Contents

Chapter 1
Fifty Years of the Philosophy and Medicine Book Series

Lisa M. Rasmussen and Søren Holm

1.1 Genesis and Purpose of the Series

The Philosophy and Medicine series was conceived by H. Tristram Engelhardt, Jr. (then at the University of Texas Medical Branch in Galveston, Texas) and Stuart F. Spicker (then at the University of Connecticut Health Center in Farmington, Connecticut) to contribute to the growing discussions of ethical and philosophical issues in the practice of medicine. It arose in the years when the United States was struggling with definitions of brain death and issues in end of life care; addressing violations of human subjects in medical research revealed in the USPHS Tuskegee Study; and witnessing the birth of what would come to be known as "bioethics."[1] This genesis is clear in the first promotional pamphlet for the series:

> The series Philosophy and Medicine has as its focus the basic conceptual foundation of these often divergent disciplines. The recent advances by medical science have caused many basic concepts to be re-examined, including the value of human life, when the life of a person begins and ends, the rights of physicians and patients, etc. As a result, widespread discussions on various levels of seriousness have begun concerning issues in medical ethics or bioethics. This series will examine the conceptual background in terms of which ques-

[1] Indeed, the series and its genesis warrants a mention in *The Birth of Bioethics*, one of the first histories of the field: "With…Stuart Spicker…[Tris Engelhardt, Jr.] initiated a long-lasting series of conferences on medicine and philosophy, which has produced an impressive series of volumes" (Jonsen 1998, 82).

L. M. Rasmussen (✉)
Department of Philosophy, University of North Carolina at Charlotte, Charlotte, NC, USA
e-mail: lrasmuss@charlotte.edu

S. Holm
School of Law, University of Manchester, Manchester, UK
e-mail: soren.holm@manchester.ac.uk

L. M. Rasmussen, S. Holm (eds.), *50 Years of Philosophy and Medicine*,
Philosophy and Medicine 150, https://doi.org/10.1007/978-3-031-95175-6_1

> tions in medical ethics can best be assayed. Though each volume of this series will attend to issues in medical ethics, these issues have been placed within much broader analyses of philosophical issues and problems in medicine and the biomedical sciences.
>
> Each volume has as its focus a different element of the conceptual background of medicine, ranging from the nature of explanation in medicine and the indebtedness of theories in medicine to value judgments, to the ways in which different construals of the mind-body problem affect modern understanding of neurology, neurophysiology, and neuro-surgery, and the meaning of such crucial concepts as mental health, mental illness, and clinical judgment.
>
> Moreover, starting with volume three, volumes in the series will from time to time include philosophers, physicians, historians of medicine, legal scholars, and social and behavioral scientists. The essays are collected with a general readership in philosophy, medicine, and the biomedical sciences in mind and offer a quality and depth of interchange among philosophers, physicians, and biomedical scientists of a wide-ranging scope, unique in the literature.
>
> The volumes include the edited proceedings of a series of trans-disciplinary symposia on philosophy and medicine held at various medical schools and universities.

Throughout its 50-year, 150-volume history, the series has remained committed to the basic tenets expressed at its birth: exploring the conceptual and ethical space between medicine and philosophy as it manifests in our world. This has resulted in a substantial focus on clinical practice; end-of-life issues such as brain death, physician-assisted death, and palliative care; conception and personhood; and the history of medical ethics. The first volume, published in 1975, was *Evaluation and Explanation in the Biomedical Sciences*, edited by series editors Engelhardt and Spicker,[2] and the next few volumes similarly focused on philosophy, medicine, and conceptual issues. But already by the 4th and 5th volumes, the series had branched into mental health and mental illness, and brought law and policy considerations to bear. Over time, the series also came to include issues in more contemporary areas, such as disability studies; gender and sexuality; and non-ideal theory in bioethics. Four subseries focusing on Asian Studies in Bioethics; Classics of Medical Ethics; Catholic Studies in Bioethics; and European Studies in Bioethics were born in later years as scholarship in these areas grew.

The series' 50 years have seen a progression of publishers (from Reidel to Kluwer to Springer to Springer Nature), a profound shift in how scholars access, produce, and disseminate knowledge, and the creation of radical new technologies like genetic engineering and AI that are already reshaping medicine in ways that demand philosophical and ethical reflection. A series like *Philosophy and Medicine* is more important than ever to host scholarship that helps us grapple with these changes.

[2] A little-known fact about this volume is that the conference that gave rise to it earned a "Golden Fleece" award in 1976 from Senator William Proxmire, "[f]or grants to well-heeled doctors, lawyers, and school administrators to attend tuition-free, vacation-like, month-long humanistic bull sessions at some of the choicest university waterholes in the country" (https://content.wisconsinhistory.org/digital/collection/proxmire/id/24). See McCullough (2015), footnote 1, for additional details about Texas-size roaches in the hotel rooms.

We are privileged and proud to reflect on the 50th year of the series with this 150th volume. Below, we reflect on the range of the series and canvass the contributions to the volume. In the process, we have been struck anew by the founding editors' foresight in creating a space for frank, civil, and rigorous discourse about some of the most pressing issues in medicine. We hope that in another 50 years, future editors will be able to say that we successfully stewarded that responsibility.

1.2 Contributions

1.2.1 Part One: Philosophy and Medicine

Medicine as a science and practice raises a number of philosophical questions that are not primarily ethical questions, although the answers to some of these questions may have ethical implications or be important premises in ethical arguments. These philosophical questions form the core of philosophy of medicine. Questions that have been extensively discussed in the series include 1) the nature and definition of concepts such as health, disease, illness, and disability; 2) the classification of diseases; 3) the nature of diagnostic reasoning; 4) the role of evidence in medical decision-making; and 5) the role and importance of phenomenology for a proper understanding of what it means to be healthy or ill. The prominence of each set of questions have waxed and waned over time, but all are still areas of active scholarly enquiry.

There has also been discussion of a meta-question, i.e., whether the philosophy of medicine actually exists as an academic field of inquiry. The agonising over this meta-question has at least partly been prompted by the perceived comparative difference in the success of bioethics and of philosophy of medicine as the fields have developed since the late 1960s.

In this volume Bjørn Hofmann and Mary Ann Gardell Cutter both discuss the developments in the analysis of the concepts of health and disease and their cognate concepts such as illness and malady.

Hofmann takes a paper on the concepts of health and disease by H. Tristram Engelhardt in the first volume in the series as his point of departure (Engelhardt Jr 1975). This paper has been cited more than 400 times and is rightly seen as one of the foundational papers in the debate about how we should understand these two concepts. Hofmann traces the debate forward and shows that there are still a number of open questions, and that new scientific developments often create new angles on the old debates, AI being the latest example. He concludes that:

> There is fair agreement that the concepts of health and disease are normative in some sense. However, what kind of norms (biological, social, cultural etc.) is contested. I have tried to show how a range of various types of values are involved in defining, classifying, and assigning health and disease. I have also pointed to a connection between facts and values in the realm of health and disease. Hence, I think there are good reasons to argue that health and disease are value-laden, but that more work is needed to clarify their value formation.

> While the literature is not clear on what kind of concepts health and disease are, it is fair to say that their extension is so diverse, that it is difficult to cover with one intension. The multifactoriality, multidimensionality, and heterogeneity of (health and) disease that Engelhardt referred to makes it difficult to capture and define the concepts according to standard criteria for definitions in one "homogenous concept" (Engelhardt Jr 1975).

We have paired Hofmann's article with a reprint of the Engelhardt paper he discusses, "The Concepts of Health and Disease."

Cutter provides an overview of the work on philosophy of medicine published in the series in the first part of her paper and argues that the unique contribution of the series is that:

> ... while the trends in contemporary medicine are to prioritize biomedical ethics over philosophy of medicine and to offer local perspectives, the Philosophy and Medicine Series has championed conceptual philosophical analysis of the claims and assumptions that frame medicine and clinical practice on a global scale. Authors in the series lay out the terrain of select issues and, when appropriate, develop the connections among the metaphysical, epistemological, and axiological dimensions of the issues set within social contexts. That is, they probe "what is…?," "how do we know…?," and "how do we value….?" in medicine, then or now, and here or there.

In the second part of her paper Cutter reflects on her own work over many years on the concept of disease, and the use of that concept in bioethics, health care, and health policy. She argues strongly that the monograph offers an opportunity for a different kind of in-depth engagement with a topic than the typical academic journal article, and that we need to keep both forms of academic publishing alive. She also shows that the philosophy of medicine provides important conceptual clarifications and premises to arguments in bioethics and health care. One of her examples related to breast cancer:

> The metaphysical, epistemological, and evaluative dimensions of disease within social contexts are not separate and distinct, but rather frame and limit each other (Cutter 2018, Ch. 6). Facts are method-ladened, the fact/method dyads are evaluative, and the fact/method/value triads are socially framed. In classifying breast cancer, for instance, a decision has to be made regarding how many cells with deviant changes of a certain kind in the biopsied breast tissue must be present before the cells are labeled as "carcinoma" or "cancer." An explanation is given about the relation between the mutating cells and breast cancer classifications and descriptions. To be too liberal in classifying cells as "cancer" will lead to unnecessary treatment, which harms patients, undermines patient autonomy, and wastes resources. To be too conservative in the classification will lead to delayed treatment, which leads to increased pain and suffering, as well as unnecessary deaths among women. On this view, the lines among "benign," "suspicious," and "cancer," as well as Stage 0 through 4 in breast cancer classification, are in part discovered and in part created. The lines among who gets clinical care and who does not, and who lives and who dies, are in part discovered and in part created. They involve explicit and implicit appeals to fact/method/value triads within social frames of reference.

In the final part of her paper Cutter provides some thoughts about how philosophy of medicine might fruitfully develop and draws particular attention to the work on 'intersectionality' in feminist theory. Taking the COVID-19 pandemic and the many types of discrimination and injustice it brought to the surface as an example, she argues convincingly that we need more philosophical work on a truly intersectional account of disease.

Fredrik Svenaeus analyses the importance of philosophical phenomenology to the philosophy of medicine taking at his point of departure Kay Toombs' magisterial and partly autobiographical book *The Meaning of Illness: A Phenomenological Account of the Different Perspectives of Physician and Patient* (Volume 42 in the P&M series). In the first part of his paper Svenaeus explicates Toombs' phenomenology of illness and traces her use of insights from four prominent phenomenologists in the continental tradition Edmund Husserl, Alfred Schutz, Jean-Paul Sartre, and Maurice Merleau-Ponty. The second part of the paper then moves on to show how analyses inspired by other phenomenologists, including Martin Heidegger, Hans-Georg Gadamer, and Medard Boss, can illuminate our understanding of the experience of being ill. Svenaeus argues that:

> The point of phenomenological approaches to medicine is to give a general characteristic of health and illness and provide a vocabulary with the aid of which one can talk about different illnesses and different ill persons and, in each case, be able to understand why and how *this* person is ill. However, this does not mean that all phenomenology can give us is good descriptions of what different individuals experience. The phenomenological description aims at uncovering necessary features of the meaning-patterns structuring our life. What breaks down in illness are the precisely the meaning-patterns of being-*in*-the-world, the way we inhabit the world through our attuned, understanding activities. The unhomelikeness of illness is consequently a certain form of senselessness, an attunement of, for instance, disorientedness, helplessness, resistance, and despair. To understand this predicament and find ways of making life less unhomelike for ill persons is the mission of healthcare practitioners.

The chapter by Søren Holm tackles the meta-question about the existence of philosophy of medicine as a proper field of inquiry. In 1992 Arthur Caplan argued that philosophy of medicine does not exist as an academic field (Caplan 1992). Caplan claimed that:

> In order to constitute a field, an inquiry must be well-integrated with other cognate inquiries and disciplines, have an established canon of key books, textbooks, anthologies and articles, and a set of distinctive and defining problems. The philosophy of medicine as it currently exists fails to satisfy these criteria and, thus, fails to exist as a field of inquiry. (Caplan 1992, p. 67)

Holm provides an overview of current activity in philosophy of medicine, including in the P&M series, and shows that Caplan's conclusion is not justified. Philosophy of medicine as it is currently practised had a set of distinctive and defining problems. It has an established canon, and it is integrated with other cognate inquiries and disciplines to the extent that should be expected in relation to a relatively small academic area. Compared to bioethics, philosophy of medicine is still a much smaller field of inquiry, but it exists and is in relatively good health.

1.2.2 Part Two: The Subseries of Philosophy and Medicine

In the 1990s, four separate P&M subseries were initiated: European Studies, Classics in Medical Ethics, Catholic Bioethics, and Asian Bioethics. Together these produced nearly two dozen volumes in the series, enabling scholarly discussion of important areas in bioethics. While for practical reasons the subseries have been dissolved, additional volumes in these subareas have continued to be published, and will be published in the future as part of the main series.

The past subseries editors have taken this opportunity to reflect back on the subseries' histories and contributions. Robert Baker starts this section out with a look back at the "Classics in Medical Ethics" subseries that aimed to bring important historical work in philosophy and medicine back into print, together with scholarly commentaries. The subseries was born from two conferences on the historical development of medical ethics in Britain and America, funded by the Wellcome Trust. After that, other classics were republished, including work by John Gregory, Elisha Bartlett, Michael Ryan, Sir Kenneth Mellanby, and Thomas Percival. The subseries also came to focus on translations into English of important work by Michael Goldberg and Rudolf Ramm.

In "The Catholic Studies in Bioethics Subseries," past subseries Editor Christopher Tollefsen traces four different aims for the subseries' founding: it provided a way to preserve scholarship that might otherwise be lost; to maintain a voice for Catholic bioethics in a field that had taken a sharply secular turn away from more Catholic beginnings; to put Catholic bioethics in dialogue with contemporary bioethics; and to "bring the resources of the Catholic tradition to bear on emerging issues" in medicine. Tollefsen ends his essay by pointing at the success of the final subseries volume (edited by Jason Eberl) in addressing these aims. It is a pleasure to note that a follow-up to that volume is already underway, maintaining the subseries' presence.

Dawei Pan and past subseries Editor Ruiping Fan canvass the Asian Subseries' history in "The Place of the Family in East Asian Bioethics." Drawing on the work of anthropologist Clifford Geertz, they argue that the volumes in this subseries can be viewed through Geertz's lenses of "pilgrim" and "cartographer." Pilgrims have an identity and view the world from that perspective, while cartographers attempt to depict what they see more objectively. Pan and Fan argue that in the subseries, each author faces the "pilgrim" question of how to establish their "Asian" identity, from which one can present and argue for a situated perspective on bioethical issues by "finding one's own voice" and "making a trenchant stand." The "cartographer" role requires reporting accurately the evidence for or against the existence of particular Asian perspectives within a particular context. Just as Tollefsen pointed out in one of the Catholic subseries' aims of putting Catholic and other moral frameworks in dialogue, Pan and Fan argue that the Asian subseries "is successful in delineating what happens when global bioethical ideas and practices diffuse into the cultural and institutional contexts of East Asian societies, which are deeply influenced by Confucian perspectives on the family, social justice, and morality."

1.2.3 Part Three: Selected Topics and Reprints From the Series' History

We also invited authors who have been connected with the series to reflect back on work in the series that has been important or formative for them. Micah Hester starts this section with "Lost in Translation: How 1979 Proved Pivotal for Bioethics and Why We Need a Narrative Account of Morality in Medicine." He argues that while the articulation of the famous four principles of bioethics was significant for the advancement of the field of bioethics, it did not come without cost. The codification of Principlism created a lingua franca in bioethics, and as Hester points out, "[f]ast forwarding nearly 50 years later, there is hardly any healthcare professional, trainee, student who has not heard about the 3–4 basic bioethical principles…" But with any such encapsulation, there is always a signal loss; for the sake of ease, dissemination, and simplification, important subtleties and foundational tenets are flattened or rendered invisible.

Hester revisits two important early essays in the series by physicians who show how the art and science of medicine can inform medical ethics. He argues not that these accounts should replace Principlism, but rather that they, too, contribute in important ways to the field of clinical ethics. As he summarizes one key difference, "[i]n both Pellegrino's and Cassell's accounts, the argument for professional practice (habit) development requires a rich understanding of patients as both the everyday people they are and the patients they see themselves to be. Such a robust approach to the medical practice, which is the groundwork for the ethical landscape of medicine, is not to be found in the early editions of the Principles." Contemporary Principlism typically interprets this as "respect for autonomy," but as Hester points out, that is not the same as the richer understanding advanced by Pellegrino and Cassell.

We pair Hester's chapter with a reprint of the two classic chapters from the series that Hester focuses on: Edmund D. Pellegrino's "Anatomy of a Clinical Judgment: Some Notes on Right Reason and Right Action," and Eric J. Cassell's chapter "The Subjective in Clinical Judgment," both from volume 6 of the series, *Clinical Judgment*.

Jason Eberl similarly focuses on an early topic in the P&M history: brain death. As Eberl points out, the series' first volume on the topic appeared in 1988 and responded to the US President's Commission report on brain death and its legislation. Subsequent controversies in brain death led to another volume in 2000. Eberl himself reflects on various approaches to the definition of death, and brain death in particular, lucidly outlining the central tenets and areas of disagreement. By itself, this outline provides an excellent overview the field for anyone trying to understand just where the disagreements stand. In addition, however, Eberl advances his own arguments for the retention of the definition of brain death as the true death of the person, based on an understanding of the brain as a true integrator of the body.

The Philosophy of Medicine book series remains committed to the careful and rigorous discussion of new and persisting issues in the field. What the next fifty years will bring depends on current and future scholars, and the perspectives they will share with us in this series.

References

Caplan, Arthur L. 1992. Does the Philosophy of Medicine Exist? *Theoretical Medicine* 13 (1): 67–77.

Cutter, Mary Ann G. 2018. *Thinking Through Breast Cancer: A Philosophical Exploration of Diagnosis, Treatment, and Survival*. New York: Oxford University Press.

Engelhardt, H., Jr. 1975. The Concepts of Health and Disease. In *Evaluation and Explanation in the Biomedical Sciences*, ed. H. T. Engelhardt Jr. and S. Spicker. Dordrecht: Reidel.

Jonsen, Albert R. 1998. The Birth of Bioethics. New York: Oxford University Press.

McCullough, Laurence B. 2015. Two Score Years Ago. In *At the Foundations of Bioethics and Biopolitics: Critical Essays on the Thought of H. Tristram Engelhardt, Jr*, ed. L. M. Rasmussen, A. S. Iltis, and M. C. Cherry. Dordrecht: Springer.

Part I
Philosophy of Medicine

Chapter 2
On the Concepts of Health and Disease

Bjørn Hofmann

In the very first edition of this book series of *Philosophy and Medicine* Tristam Engelhardt Jr. wrote a seminal chapter *The concepts of health and disease* (Engelhardt 1975) in which he elaborated on three crucial issues: (1) the ontology of health and disease, (2) the evaluative status of the concepts, and (3) the relationship between them. While many scholarly discussions have taken place in the 50 years since the publication, and progress has been made, the key issues are still up for grabs. In this chapter, I will address six key questions: (i) what are the things called health and disease? (ii) To what extent and how are the concepts of health and disease value-laden? (iii) What kind of concepts are health and disease? (iv) What is the role of models of health and disease? (v) What is the relationship between health and disease? (vi) and what is the relationship between disease and diagnosis? To address these questions, I will use the literature that has been published since Engelhardt's chapter.

2.1 What Are These Things Called Health and Disease? The Ontological Question

The ontological status of the phenomena referred to when using the words "health" and "disease" has been debated since antiquity. The key issue is whether the phenomena of health and disease are given by nature or culture (or both). Most people

B. Hofmann (✉)
Center for Medical Ethics, University of Oslo, Oslo, Norway

Institute for the Health Sciences, Norwegian University of Science and Technology, Gjøvik, Norway
e-mail: b.m.hofmann@medisin.uio.no

L. M. Rasmussen, S. Holm (eds.), *50 Years of Philosophy and Medicine*,
Philosophy and Medicine 150, https://doi.org/10.1007/978-3-031-95175-6_2

(and even many scholars) will agree that a tangible lump on a person's neck is a phenomenon in nature. However, whether we classify the lump as a disease (e.g., in terms of the disease type cancer) may well depend on a range of different social aspects.

This has divided scholars in the philosophy of medicine in two main camps: *Naturalists* claiming that health and/or disease are given by natural phenomena (Bechtel 1985; Guerrero 2010; Hershenov 2020; Khushf 2007; Kingma 2014; Nordenfelt 2013; Sholl and Okholm 2021; Veit 2021; Hausman 2012, 2014) and *normativists* arguing that they are determined by social phenomena (King 1954; Sedgwick 1973; Cooper 2002; Kukla 2014), e.g., social norms. Additionally, a third camp has emerged, claiming that health and disease are given both by natural and social phenomena, also known as *hybridists* (Powell and Scarffe 2019; Wakefield 2007). As such, the ontological debate has departed somewhat from Engelhardts's origin, where the phenomena of disease were (i) etiologically differentiated entities, (ii) (physiological) changes, or (iii) characteristic patterns.

2.1.1 Things, Changes, or Patterns?

Engelhardts' analysis builds on the ancient differentiation between "ontological conceptions of disease" and "physiological conceptions of disease" (Hofmann 2001b). According to the first, diseases are entities given by an underlying (etiological) reality. On the other hand, the physiological conception views disease as change or deviance from a norm or standard. While the first can be traced back to the Knidian medical school in antiquity, according to which diseases existed as classifiable entities, the second has been connected the Coan school of medicine (i.e., the Hippocratic) and theories of homeostasis (Hofmann 2001b). Engelhardt connects the division between ontological and physiological conceptions to the realist and anti-realist positions in the philosophy of science.

Interestingly, the physiological conceptions of disease has obtained new attention through the biomarkerization of medicine, where biomarkers come to monitor changes in a broad range of biological conditions (Metzler 2010; Boenink and van der Molen 2024). Correspondingly, the ontological perspective has revived its relevance as precision medicine has fuelled the belief in etiologically understandings of disease (Vogt and Hofmann 2022).

According to the third type of disease ontology mentioned in Engelhardt's seminal chapter, disease is given by specific characteristic patterns. "the constellation or cluster of the signs and symptoms which form the character of a disease" (Engelhardt 1975). While this non-reified conception of disease ontology has gained less scholarly attention since Engelhardt's publication in 1975, it still appears to have appeal amongst clinicians.

Although medicine is a wholeheartedly pragmatic endeavour quite independent of ontological preconceptions, clinicians tend to think that diseases exist independent of shifting human classification systems and that disease in general has some characteristic pattern making it object-like (Burns 1975). What characterizes the "object of disease" or "the thing called disease" is a set of characteristic symptoms and signs (Nordenfelt 1995). These may be given as the sum of specific properties (in a Russellian sense), as the polarizing characteristic connecting diverse phenomena together (in a phenomenological, Husserlian sense), or as ideas (in a Platonic sense).

Since Engelhardt's analysis, much attention has been given to health and disease as socially constructed phenomena, especially as they are imbued with social values (see below). However, with some exceptions (Conrad and Barker 2010; Martin and Peterson 2009), few scholars have been explicit on what is socially constructed (Hacking 1991) when it comes to health and disease. One reason why less efforts have been made to clarify exactly which norms form our conceptions of health and disease (and how) may be that the concepts lose their demarcation power when becoming culturally contextual. Using a socially constructed concept to differentiate socially conceived situations may not be socially efficient or convincing.

Hence, after much more than 50 years of fierce debates, there is no general agreement on the ontological status of health and disease. While the ontological landscape is divided into naturalists, normativists, and hybridists, many theories of health and disease include basic phenomena, such as wellbeing, pain, suffering, (dys)function and/or (in)capacity and/or (in)ability, as well as some epistemic (identifying and/or explanatory) relationship to biological and/or mental phenomena. However, exactly which of these phenomena make up health and disease, and how, is still up for grabs.

2.2 Is It Value Neutral or Value-Laden?

The ontological question of *what health and disease are* has been intertwined and sometimes mixed up with the question of whether the concepts are *value neutral or value-laden* (Elselijn Kingma 2017; Broadbent 2019; De Vreese 2017; DeVito 2000; Kingma 2014; Nordenfelt 2007; Goosens 1980). This may be because naturalists tend to claim that health and disease are value neutral phenomena (and concepts) while normativists have claimed that they are value-laden. For example, Sedgwick clearly claims that "[t]he medical enterprise is from its inception value-loaded; it is not simply an applied biology, but a biology applied in accordance with the dictates of social interest." (Sedgwick 1973) Similarly, Sade argues that "[d]isease can be understood as a biologically based value concept" (Sade 1995) while Reznek explains that the "concept of disease is a normative or evaluative concept. Judging that same condition as a disease is to judge that the person with that condition is less able to lead a good or worthwhile life. And since this latter judgement is a normative one, to judge that some condition is a disease is to make a normative judgement" (Reznek 1987).

Naturalists, like Boorse (1975, 1977, 2011, 2014), have been challenged to explain how nature can set the limits for disease, e.g., with respect to cut-off values, thresholds, and reference classes for a wide range of diseases. According to this "line-drawing problem" (Rogers and Walker 2017; Hofmann 2021) the challenge is to show how the norms (and limits) are set by nature and not by culture (e.g., out of social interests to help people). To avoid the problem Boorse refers to "nonnormative norms" where the norms of nature are to sustain survival and reproduction, and where anything obstructing this is of negative value (Boorse 1975). Others have referred to biological norms (Lindstrøm 2012), functional efficiency (Hausman 2014; Cooper 2017), and biological normativity (Veit 2021; Griffiths and Matthewson 2018; Matthewson and Griffiths 2017). Nonetheless, the question of how nature sets the limits for health and disease (and between them) has not yet found a general and convincing argument (to many scholars).

Accordingly, social norms and values have not yet been ruled out (even from naturalist accounts) (Veit 2021), and the limit between biological and social norms are neither sharp nor clarified. There appear to be at least two reasons why the issue of value has not been settled during these passing 50 years since Engelhardt's claim that both health and disease are valueladen. The first is that we have not been specific to what types of values health and disease are "laden with." That is, the value play of health and disease has not been sufficiently elucidated. The second is that the relationship between facts and values has not been adequately clarified.

2.2.1 Types of Values in Health and Disease

Disease is generally considered to be bad, while health is good. As Engelhardt pointed out "[t]he concept [of health] is both aesthetic and ethical, suggesting what is beautiful and what is good. By terming something diseased, one indicates that the state of affairs is both naturally ugly as well as one that imposes some obligations and relieves others" (Engelhardt 1975). While health often is considered to be an intrinsic value, disease is less often so. This may be because disease is multivalent, e.g., by also having positive values. See below.

The value of health and disease is reflected in etymology. Terms like "dis-ease", dys-function, and dis-ability contain a (d)evaluative "dis-" or "dys-" of something valued (ease, ability, function). The term health stems from Old English hǣlth, whole or hale (free from disease or infirmity; robust; vigorous). The negative value of disease is often referred to in terms of harm. However, what counts as harm is still debated, e.g., whether it is pain, reduced function, suffering (Hofmann 2024), disability, loss of freedom or autonomy (Engelhardt and Wildes 1995; Tristram Engelhardt Jr 1973), or the setback of interests (Feinberg 1989).

Moreover, health and disease incite moral appeals. Disease incites a moral appeal in terms of an impetus to avoid, reduce, or eliminate it, while health may incite a moral impetus to ascertain and promote it. Moreover, there are a range of arguments for the similarities and differences in the moral appeal between health and disease (Hofmann 2023b) and the related concepts of wellbeing and suffering (Hofmann 2024). These issues have substantial ethical and practical implications for priority

Table 2.1 Overview of how disease gives and takes away rights and obligations (to and from individuals)

	Rights	Obligations	
Takes away	Driver's license, parental responsibility, freedom (freedom of movement, from coercion)	Work, social moral responsibility, criminal liability (in case of lack of sanity)	**Frees from**
Gives	Sickness benefit, right to health care, social benefits	Seek help, avoid infection and infecting others	**Assigns**

setting in healthcare and is one reason why the issue of valueladenness is so important (and heatedly debated). See also below.

In addition to moral values and appeals, health and especially disease have a range moral functions. Whether you are healthy or have a disease gives you a series of rights and obligations – or takes them away. As summarized in Table 2.1, being diseased gives your rights to health care, sickness benefit, and other social benefits. Conversely, disease can also take away rights, such as having a driver's license, having parental responsibility, or being allowed to move freely (e.g., in case of having a contagious infection). Disease can also free from social obligations, such as work, but also from criminal liability (in case of insanity). Conversely, disease may assign obligations, such as the duty to seek help or avoid infecting others. These moral functions can explain why it is crucial to clarify the valueladenness of (health and especially) disease.

Disease also has epistemic value (Stempsey 1999). Knowing that a person has a disease explains why the person is not able to behave as wanted or expected. It reduces both professional and personal uncertainty. Correspondingly, disease has a practical value, being action guiding both socially with respect to the rights and obligations mentioned above, and professionally as specific diseases give guidance for particular actions, such as diagnostics, treatment, and palliation.

Disease also has a range of social values. E.g., diseases form prestige hierarchies according to which diseases that can be connected to specific organs (that are placed high up in the body), that are acute, can be detected and treated with advanced technologies, occurring in young people have high prestige (Album et al. 2017; Album and Westin 2008) and conversely. Correspondingly, diseases can be stigmatized and stigmatizing as (some) diseases are related to personal identity. However, diseases can also give social status in particular cases.[1]

As Engelhardt (1975) and others (Jutel and Buetow 2007) have pointed out, health and disease also have aesthetic value: health is beauty and disease is ugly. This may have a range of evolutionary explanations, as ugly is framed by what is dangerous. However, the aesthetic connotations of health and disease may also induce social injustice (Hofmann 2023c).

Moreover, the moral functions (mentioned above) make what disease is, and what is considered to be disease, important moral issues to control. Several stakeholders have gone to great efforts to expand disease (Hofmann 2018, 2019b) as well

[1] This goes back to ancient Greeks calling epilepsy "the sacred disease".

as health (Hofmann 2023a; Schroeder 2013). At the same time, others try to restrict them (Giles 2014; Beek et al. 2016). Accordingly, defining, classifying, and assigning disease gives substantial social power (Farmer 1999; Paul 2003; Rose 2009). This is well demonstrated in the vast and vivid debates of the revision of the classification systems, such as the ICD and DSM as well as in the attribution of certain diseases.

Additionally, disease is (dis)valued differently from the perspective of the person experiencing the illness, from the professional diagnosing and treating the disease, and from the perspective of society attributing a sick role (sickness) to the person (Hofmann 2016; Hofmann and Eriksen 2001).

Table 2.2 summarizes various types of values involved in defining, classifying, and assigning health and disease. Again (and surprisingly), the value issues with health appears to be less controversial and there are several suggestions of how health relates to values, e.g., to human capabilities (Richardson 2016; Venkatapuram 2009).

This overview is by no means exhaustive or exclusive as disease also has been considered to be of positive value, e.g., at the end of life: "Pneumonia may well be called the friend of the aged. Taken off by it in an acute, short, not often painful illness, the old man escapes those 'cold gradations of decay' so distressing to himself and to his friends" (Osler 1916). Correspondingly, there has been a strong cognitive association between morality and health and sinfulness and disease (Lakoff and Johnson 1999; Martin 2006).

2.2.2 *Valuing Facts and Facting Values*

The close moral connotations of health and disease has resulted in a strong interconnection between ontology and ethics. As we have seen, when something is considered to be disease, there appears to be a strong moral appeal to help the person to avoid, reduce, or remove it (Hofmann 2023b). On the other hand, when something is considered to be bad, there is a strong tendency to make it a disease, i.e., to conceive of the phenomena to be disease. For example, when we want to help people with their grief – we tend to make grief a disease (Wakefield 2013). Figure 2.1 tries to illustrate this relationship between facts and values related to disease.

There are of course many reasons for this, e.g., that the healthcare system is an institution that is considered to be successful in removing socially considered "bads." However, philosophically this is problematic, as it involves reasoning both from *is* to *ought* and from *ought* to *is* (Hofmann 2022a).

Table 2.2 Overview of various types of values involved in defining, classifying, and assigning health and disease

Type	Explanation	Examples and comments
Moral value	*Disease* is bad (dis-ease) and health is good *Health* is often considered to be an intrinsic (positive) value, while disease a negative value (but not always)	This is reflected in the etymology: dis-ease, dys-function, and dis-ability having (d) evaluative prefixes, like "dis-" or "dys-" and health stemming from Old English hǣlth, whole or hale
Moral appeal	*Disease* incites moral impetus to avoid, reduce, or eliminate disease. *Health* incites a moral appeal to promote it.	Pain and suffering from disease urges individuals and professionals to help and wellbeing urges to promote health (at least according to classical consequentialism). See Hofmann (2023b, 2024) for a discussion on this
Moral function (of disease)	Attributing rights Freeing from duties Removing or restricting rights Attributing accountability	Patients have the right to attention and care Patients are freed from the duty to work (sick leave) Persons are freed from moral and legal rights and responsibilities (drivers license, legal accountability)
Epistemic value (of disease)	Knowing why a person is not able to behave as wanted or expected	Reduces professional and personal uncertainty Provides explanation for social role attribution
Practical value (of disease)	Action guiding	Professionals know what to do for specific diseases Social institutions are guided in attributions of rights
The social value of disease	*Diseases* have prestige and social status The moral functions (above) make it interesting for stakeholders to control (expand) what is considered to be disease Defining and assigning disease gives power	Prestige hierarchies of disease can result in stigmatization, discrimination, and injustice Expanding the concept of disease may be helpful and harmful (overdiagnosis, overtreatment) There is power in defining, classifying diseases and in applying classifications
Values related to different perspectives on disease	Patients experience and dis-value disease differently from professionals and society and social institutions	Patients disvalue illness Professionals attribute (dis)value to various diseases Society disvalues sickness in assigning sick role
Aesthetic values	*Health* is considered to be beautiful *Disease* is considered to be ugly	Beauty is associated with good and ugly is associated with bad or dangerous resulting in potential "aesthetic injustice"

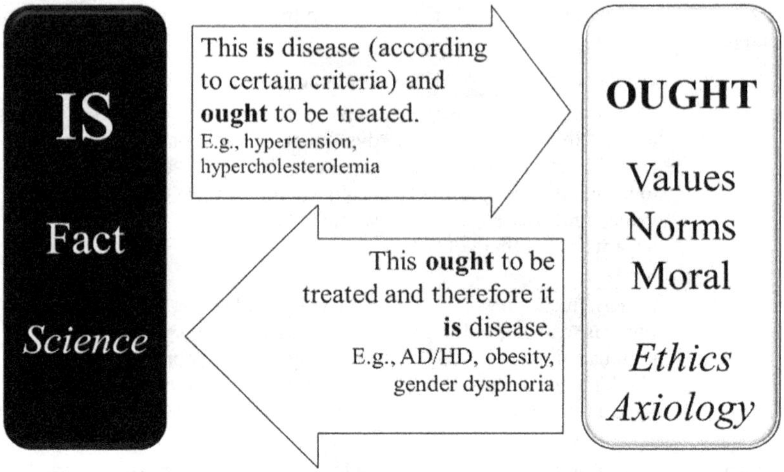

Fig. 2.1 Illustration of the reciprocal relationship between facts and values related to disease

Table 2.3 Four positions on the value-relationship of health and disease, positions (according to Broadbent (2019)), and some authors who have described or represent the positions

	Objective	Subjective
Value-neutral	*Naturalists*: Health and disease are objective facts in the world independent of (social) values. (Value-independent realism, Boorse)	Health and disease are something existing through our perception, i.e., because we recognize it (value-independent anti-realism, Broadbent)
Value-laden	Values are facts Health and disease are facts that include objective values (value-dependent realism, Stempsey, Neo-Aristotelianism, Kingma)	*Normativists*: Health and disease are value-related concepts that depend on human (subjective) values (value-dependent anti-realism, Cooper, Sedgwick)

2.2.3 *Is It Subjective or Objective?*

Connected to the debate on whether health and disease are value-laden or not, there is a discussion of whether health and disease are something subjective or objective. Naturalists typically claim that health and disease are objective while normativists typically tend to claim that they are subjective phenomena. However, as illustrated in Table 2.3, it is possible to claim that health and disease can be value-neutral and subjective, and that they can be value-laden and objective (Kingma 2017; Broadbent 2019).

In sum, the relationship between health, disease, and value is a complex one and has not yet found any coherent and unifying solution. One reason for this may be that there has been too little clarity on what is meant with "value" and too poor differentiation between the various types of values involved in the different debates (Hofmann et al. 2018).

2.3 What Kind of Concepts Are Health and Disease?

As also becomes clear from the review of the literature, the ontological question of what health and disease *is* has not only been intertwined (and confused) with the ethical issue of good and bad. Ontological issues (on the phenomena of health and disease) have been entangled with conceptual issues, belonging to semantics, linguistics, or philosophy of language. Moreover, it is not always clear what kind of concepts health and disease are.

2.3.1 Category, Type, and Token

One challenge in conceptual debates about (health and) disease is clarity on the subject matter. It is unclear what is discussed: the general category of disease, disease entities, or instances of disease. The reason for this is that disease entities and specific disease cases are widely used as examples in the scholarly debates on the general category of disease (Gagné-Julien 2024; Burgess et al. 2020). However, instances of disease (token) is a matter for diagnostics, while disease entities (type) is an issue for nosology, and the general category of disease concerns philosophy (Sadegh-Zadeh 2008). Increased clarity on this can clearly improve future scholarly work.

2.3.2 Vague, Fuzzy, or (Proto-)Typical?

Other debates have been about what kind of concepts health and disease are: classical, vague, prototypical etc. Traditionally, scholars have tried to define the general categories (concepts) of health and disease by searching for a set of essential features or criteria that are common to all instances of health and disease respectively. If a specific case of disease (token) or disease entity (type) is possessing a series of defining features, then this qualifies for falling under the general concept of disease. As stated in Plato's Meno: what makes something X, is that all cases of X have "a common nature which makes them" X (Meno 72).

However, it has been difficult to agree on such sets of essential features. As Ludwig Wittenstein pointed out: "Doctors will use names for diseases without ever deciding which phenomena should be taken as criteria and which as symptoms; and this is not necessarily a deplorable lack of clarity. For remember, we do not generally use language according to strict rules - nor have we been taught by means of strict rules. Instead, in our discussions, we constantly compare language to a calculation that takes place according to precise rules." (Wittgenstein 1958).

As a result, a series of alternatives to such classical theories of concepts have emerged. For example, it has been suggested that health and disease are vague concepts, i.e., that they elusive (Boyd 2000), or have vague or blurry boundaries (Hampton 2007; Hauswald and Keuck 2017; Hofmann 2010; Hucklenbroich 2017; Keil and Stoecker 2016; Stoecker and Keil 2016). "Vagueness generally relates to the question of whether or not, and to what degree an instance falls within a conceptual category" (Hampton 2007). Still, it is not always clear what is vague, whether it is the world itself, the concept (intension), its extension, language use, or all of these.

Relatedly, others have suggested that health and disease are fuzzy concepts, following fuzzy logic (Sadegh-Zadeh 2000; Seising 2006). Moreover, inspired by the family resemblance theory of Wittgenstein and insights in learning theory (e.g., central statistical tendency in categorization), it has been proposed that disease is a prototype concept (Bishop et al. 1987; Hampton 1995; Lalljee et al. 1993; Papa and Li 2015; Sadegh-Zadeh 2008; Wakefield 1999). Some instances are more or less prototypical for a disease type, and some disease types are more or less prototypical for disease in general.

2.3.3 Ambiguity, Heteronomy, and Complexity

Already Engelhardt, and others before him, pointed out that health and disease are ambiguous and heterogeneous concepts:

> The concepts are ambiguous, operating both as explanatory and evaluatory notions. They describe states of affairs, factual conditions, while at the same time judging them to be good or bad. … Perhaps the concept of disease indicates a family of conceptually consanguineous notions. …the concept of disease may be a basically heterogeneous concept standing for a set of phenomena collected together out of diverse social interests, not on the basis of the recognition of a natural type or a common conceptual structure.

However, how we should conceptualize this ambiguity or heteronomy is a challenging issue that has gained much attention but obtained little consensus since Engelhardt's publication. It can be argued that the very many (descriptive and prescriptive) aspects of the phenomena of health and disease make their concepts complex (Hofmann 2001a, 2010; Vandamme et al. 2013) and that we may need to differentiate in different concepts, such as disease, illness, sickness Hofmann 2016; Hofmann and Eriksen 2001), and others (Rogers and Walker 2018).

As many diseases share certain features, such as being disvalued, harmful, statistically abnormal, medically manageable, and involve dysfunction of some kind (Kingsbury and McKeown-Green 2009), it has been suggested that disease is a cluster concept, characterized by a cluster of non-necessary, but sufficient features (Walker and Rogers 2018; Stoecker and Keil 2016). Yet another approach is to conceive of health and disease as polysemic concepts, i.e., that they have more than one meaning (Gangemi et al. 2000).

Moreover, with Locke it can be argued that health and disease are "forensic concepts," or with Wieland that they are deontological concepts (Wieland 2013). One may also maintain with Hare and Williams that they are "thick concepts" that are both descriptive and prescriptive (Hare 1952, 1986) or that they are "dual character concepts" (Knobe et al. 2013). Correspondingly, health and disease can be claimed to be variable (Visser 2023), practical (van der Linden and Schermer 2022), serviceable (Kaebnick 2013), or multivalent concepts (Gerring et al. 2021; Gerring 1999).

Hence, there are many relevant and fruitful attempts to capture the fact that what falls under the concepts of health and disease is diverse. This lack of conceptual clarity is in many ways connected to the lack of ontological clearness (described above) and has fuelled the question of whether we actually need the concepts of health and disease in the first place.

If the concepts are vague, they can do little practical work, e.g., in terms of demarcation. Correspondingly, it has been argued that disease is an irrelevant (Hesslow 1993) or futile (Worrall and Worrall 2001) concept that should be abandoned in medical contexts and replaced by "biomedical states that are disvalued" (Ereshefsky 2009). The anti-psychiatry movement (Szasz 1960) has also been presented (more or less rightly) as being against disease categories in psychiatry. However, while providing relevant critiques of the efforts to provide clear and useful definitions of concepts of health and disease, the concepts have neither been abandoned nor have alternative concepts have been well established.

As little consensus has been reached on the heteronomy of the concepts of health and disease, prominent attempts have been made to make models of health and disease that are able to capture the variety of features, characteristics, or aspects.

2.4 Models of Health and Disease

The most influential model was suggested by Engel in 1977 (Engel 1977). The bio-psycho-social model is a multifaceted model that advances the interrelations between biological, psychological, and socio-environmental aspects of health and disease. It was developed and framed against a biomedical dominance, and as such has been able to broaden the scope. Figure 2.2 illustrates the model.

While there is broad agreement on the influence of the model, it has been criticized for not being evidence-based, having limited clinical and scientific value (e.g., in terms of aetiology), and having a poor philosophical foundation (Bolton and Gillett 2019; Kendler 2010). While the model has been framed to be holistic (and interdisciplinary), it can also be criticized for being reductionistic, reducing aspects of health and disease to biological, mental, and social phenomena.

Other models have evolved to address other aspects. For example, a socio-ecological framework, based on the developmental psychology Bronfenbrenner (1977), has been established for a range of areas, especially for health promotion. More narrowly, disease entity models have also been elaborated (Whitbeck 1977).

This is obviously not the place for in-depth studies of health and disease models beyond pointing out that they try to address some of the basic philosophical issues mentioned above. In particular, they try to address the multifaceted aspects of the

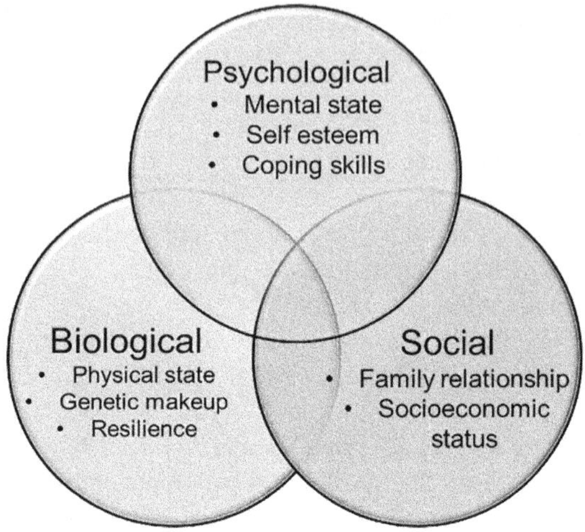

Fig. 2.2 Visualization of Engel's biopsychosocial model of health and disease

concepts and that many of them include personal, professional, societal, and environmental features.

2.5 What Is the Relationship Between Health and Disease?

One important topic that has gained somewhat less attention is the relationship between health and disease. Engelhardt points out that "health and disease are not symmetrical concepts" and that the concept of disease is a pragmatic one directed towards (the ideal of) health and that health is "a regulative ideal of autonomy". "The concept of health helps define the concept of disease by providing the telos for the medical enterprise. Disease concepts are, as has been argued, pragmatic concepts whose truth is found in action directed to the elimination of illness and toward the establishment of health" (Engelhardt 1975).

Boorse and Nordenfelt have written extensively on both concepts. According to Boorse "health is normal functioning, where the normality is statistical and the functions biological" (Boorse 1977) while disease is state of statistically species-subnormal biological functional ability, relative to sex and age (Boorse 2014). To Nordenfelt, illness (un-health and not disease) is the opposite of health, while disease is an internal process that can cause illness (Nordenfelt 1986, 1993, 1995, 2005, 2007). WHO has stated that "health is more than the absence of disease" (1946) but has not specified the relationship between the concepts and its definition of health has been more politically motivated than philosophically sound (Bickenbach 2015).

As I so far have focused more on disease than health, let me summarize some of the conceptions of health that have been prominent in the literature in Table 2.4.

Table 2.4 Overview of some prominent conceptions of health with explanations, examples, and origin

Conception of health	Explanation or example	Origin, reference
Normal functioning	(Statistically) normal functioning contributing to survival and reproduction	Boorse (1977)
Wellbeing	"a state of complete physical, mental, and social wellbeing and not merely the absence of disease or infirmity"	World Health Organization (1946)
Homeostasis, balance	Internal and external balance	Sigerist (1941), Recio (1974), Ananth (2017)
Meaning	Sense of coherence	Antonovsky (1985)
Ability	Ability to realize own goals	Pörn (1984, 1993)
	Capacity to contribute to realizing own goals	Whitbeck (1981)
	Ability to contribute to realizing vital goals (minimal happiness)	Nordenfelt (1995, 2005)
	Capabilities	Richardson (2016), Venkatapuram (2013)
Flourishing	Happiness and life satisfaction, physical and mental health, meaning and purpose, character and virtue, close social relationships, and financial and material security	VanderWeele et al. (2019)
Tolerance, margin, resilience	Ability to adapt, tolerance of change, resilience to stress	Canguilhem (1989)
Deemed healthy social construction	What the prevailing culture deems as healthy	Sharf and Vanderford (2003)

Four models of the relationship between health and disease have been identified in the literature as well as in clinical practice and in the lay population: The ideal model, the medical model, the holistic model, and the disjunctive model (Hofmann 2005).

According to *the ideal model*, you are either healthy or diseased. Health and disease are exhaustive and mutually exclusive concepts (Burns 1975). This model excludes being both healthy and diseased and being neither.

The holistic model claims that it takes more than the absence of disease to be healthy. Hence, health is the primary concept (to be defined). WHO's definition of health is but one example of this model. According to *the medical model* it takes more than the absence of health to be diseased. You need specific criteria to be diseased, and disease is the concept primarily being defined.

Both the holistic and the medical model encompass being neither healthy nor diseased, but none of them allow being both healthy and diseased. Both of these options are available in *the disjunctive model* where health and disease are opposite and partly independent concepts (Hofmann 2005).

It is interesting to notice that patients, professionals, and policy makers can apply several models, e.g., in different contexts. Moreover, it may be argued that there are

Table 2.5 Potential differences between the concepts of health and disease

	Health	Disease
Ontological	Wellbeing, pleasure, function, balance, harmony	Pain, suffering, dysfunction, dis-ability, reduced capacity
Epistemological	Physiology (partly learned through pathology)	Pathology
Nosological	No taxonomy of health	Many taxonomies of disease
Etymological	Whole, hale	Dis-ease, dys-function
Experiential	Basis for experience, enigmatic, evasive, (minimal happiness)	Experienced (pain, reduced function, ability or capacity)
Axiological (value)	Positive value (mainly)	Negative value (mainly)
Conceptual	Difficult to define Vague	(Somewhat less) Difficult to define
Practical	Difficult to operationalize	(less) Difficult to operationalize
Moral	Impetus to promote the wellbeing of others (weak)	Impetus to reduce the suffering of others (strong)

crucial differences between the phenomena of health and disease and their concepts. Table 2.5 summarizes some of these differences. For more details, see (Hofmann 2005).

2.6 What Is the Relationship Between Disease and Diagnosis and Between Health and Health Indicators?

Traditionally, diagnoses have been labels of disease, i.e., names for specific diseases. Accordingly, diagnostic manuals were taxonomies of diseases, and there was a close connection between a diagnosis and manifest (and experienced) disease. However, with great advances in science and technology it became possible to identify and label a wide range of indicators of disease, such as risk factors, precursors, and predictors (Hofmann 2018). As such indicators can be of great importance to the prevention, diagnostics, and surveillance of disease as well as assessing treatment susceptibility and progression, hey were given diagnostic names after the diseases they indicated. However, this has resulted in a looser connection between disease and diagnosis. Indicators only indicate disease, they do not verify it. Moreover, you can have a diagnosis without having a disease (as classification systems included diagnoses of conditions that were not considered to be disease). Gender incongruence is but one example (Beek et al. 2016).

Thus, diagnostic manuals are not (pure) disease taxonomies anymore. This has implications for the ethics of disease. For example, if disease is the driver of moral appeal due to its connection to pain, dysfunction, and suffering (Hofmann 2024), then diagnoses closer connected to disease should have higher priority than those who are remote or who are not connected to pain, suffering, or dysfunction, etc.

Correspondingly, various health indicators and biomarkers are used more extensively to confirm and monitor health (Sim et al. 2022; Etches et al. 2006; Levin and Bradshaw 2023). On the one hand this may contribute to operationalize the concept of health and further health measurement and management. On the other hand, it can expand the concept of health by furthering health enhancement (Hofmann 2019a).

The point here is not to enter the vast and vivid debate on indicators of health and disease, but only to indicate that technological advancements influence basic conceptual relationships in medicine, such as the one between disease and diagnosis and between health and its measures. Another interesting implication of this is that technology not only influences our concepts of health and disease (Hofmann 2017, 2001c) but also our experiences of wellbeing and illness (Hofmann and Svenaeus 2018). Correspondingly, it can be expected that science and technology will influence the social role of sickness.

2.7 Concepts – Definitions – Theories

As health and disease are crucial concept for a key institution in most societies, i.e., the healthcare system, and they have great moral and social implications in terms of attention, access to care, and resource allocation, great efforts have been made to define the concepts. A range of criteria (Nordenfelt 2005; Bjørn Morten Hofmann 2022b; Gerring 1999) and procedures (Gagné-Julien 2024; Burgess et al. 2020) have been suggested for providing robust and useful definitions of health and disease.

Some common *formal criteria* are precision, neutrality, operationality, and non-circularity. In addition, there are a wide range of *substantive* criteria, such as that definitions must refer to "real phenomena" (ontological), must be evidence-based and differentiating (epistemic), be just in attributing and revoking rights and duties (moral), must be communication-coordinating and action-guiding (practical), and express the goal of medicine (teleological criteria) (Hofmann 2022b).

One additional criterium is more contested, i.e., the criterion that the definition has to be theoretically well founded (Nordenfelt 2005; Fabrega Jr. 1976; Gannik 2002; Kovacs 1998; Nordenfelt 2000; Sade 1995; Wakefield 2014; Whitbeck 1981). Clearly, sound theories can justify definitions, but they can also generate controversies. As Kukla points out, one of the reasons why "the various attempts to define health and disease have been so unsatisfactory is that those using the notion are driven by deeply diverse theoretical and practical goals"(Kukla 2014). Table 2.6 provides an overview of selected theories of disease.

As there has been neither been agreement on theories of health and disease, nor on the definition of the concepts, it has suggested that we need to define the concept for specific (and limited) areas or purposes, such as within the field of overdiagnosis (Rogers and Walker 2018). Others have elaborated on Carnap's concept of explication (Carnap 1962) and developed what has become known as conceptual

Table 2.6 Historical overview of selected theories of disease

Theory	Time period	Conception of disease	Origin, example, scholar
Demonic	All times?	Evil spirits	Ancient Egypt
Vitalism	2000 BC	Vital principle	Ancient Egypt, Greece
Humoral pathology	400 BC–1800 AD	Imbalance of four humors	Hippocrates, Greek (Coan) medicine
Miasma	500 BC–1880 AD	Pollution through air	India, ancient Greece
Neohumoralism	1620-	Anomalies in blood	William Harvey
Stimulus-Response theory	1850-	Response to stimuli	Florence Nightingale
Germ theory Bacteriology	1850-	Bacteria	Louis Pasteur, Robert Koch
Altered anatomy	1750- 1800- 1850-	Altered organs Altered tissue Altered cells	Giovanni Morgagni Xavier Bichat Rudolph Virchow
Genetic	1980-	Genetic causes	Frederick Sanger, Kary Banks Mullis
Risk (model)	1950-	Elevated risk	Epidemiology, Disease prevention and health promotion
Bio-psycho-social (model)	1980-	Complex conception	George L. Engel
Systems biology	2000-	Interaction of genes, proteins, environment	Ludwig von Bertalanffy
Artificial Intelligence Machine Learning	2020-	Associations based on BigData analysis	Deep Medicine, Eric Topol

engineering in order to design, implement, and evaluate concepts (Burgess et al. 2020), including health and disease (Gagné-Julien 2024).

In sum, there is by now a range of definitions of health and disease, both general and specific, theory-based and empirical, value-laden and value-free, as well as theoretical and pragmatic. All have their merits and flaws, and no major consensus has been reached.

2.8 Discussion

While I have addressed several issues, many have been left out (due to lack of space). The epistemology of health and disease is but one of these, including causality and classification systems. Moreover, the concepts of health and disease change over time. People now have different diseases than before, doctors change their ideas about disease over time, and the social significance of disease alters (Jones et al. 2012). These conceptual changes are worth separate studies.

As argued, all the issues of this chapter are controversial. So is my presentation of them. There is no "view from nowhere" in debates on health and disease. Hence, my review of some of the core issues is itself open for discussion.

Additionally, each of the issues are worth books of their own. Therefore, this chapter necessarily will appear swift and superficial. However, the intention has been to provide an overview of the development and status of the topics that Engelhardt raised in his seminal chapter in 1975.

While this chapter clearly has very many references, many more are left out. My reference managing system on the topic of Disease alone has more than 1600 references, and only a few of those are included. Not citing authors and references is not due to the lack of interest or importance, but due to the scarcity of space.

2.9 Conclusion

In his seminal article, Engelhardt discussed the ontology of health and disease, the evaluative status of the concepts, and the relationship between them. In this chapter, I have tried to (narratively) review some of the discussions that have played out in the 50 years since the publication. I have done so by addressing six key questions: (i) what are the things called health and disease? (ii) to what extent and how are the concepts of health and disease value-laden? (iii) what kind of concepts are health and disease? (iv) what is the role of models of health and disease? (v) what is the relationship between health and disease? (vi) what is the relationship between disease and diagnosis? So, what are the answers to these crucial questions?

The phenomena of health and disease can be studied from a wide range of perspectives, methods, and approaches, each uncovering important aspects. So far, it has been difficult to unite these into *one thing*. As Engelhardt points out: "Diseases are, as the physiological nosologists stressed, much more complex than the easy simplicity implicit in many ontological nosologies. Diseases are, in fact, not only multifactorial, but multidimensional, involving genetic, physiological, psychological, and sociological components. .... diseases have a basically relational, not a subject (i.e., substance)-predicate (accident) nature" (Engelhardt 1975). Hence, the ontological question does not yet have a clear answer reaching adequate consensus.

There is fair agreement that the concepts of health and disease are normative in some sense. However, what kind of norms (biological, social, cultural etc.) is contested. I have tried to show how a range of various types of values are involved in defining, classifying, and assigning health and disease. I have also pointed to a connection between facts and values in the realm of health and disease. Hence, I think there are good reasons to argue that health and disease are value-laden, but that more work is needed to clarify their value formation.

While the literature is not clear on what kind of concepts health and disease are, it is fair to say that their extension is so diverse, that it is difficult to cover with one intension. The multifactoriality, multidimensionality, and heterogeneity of (health and) disease that Engelhardt referred to makes it difficult to capture and define the concepts according to standard criteria for definitions in one "homogenous concept" (Engelhardt 1975).

Corresponding to the multidimensionality of the concepts of (health and) disease, models have emerged, been applied, and critiqued. Common to many of the models is that they include personal, professional, societal, and environmental features.

For Engelhardt "[t]he concept of health helps define the concept of disease by providing the telos for the medical enterprise. … Health is the common way away from the many ways of disease." (Engelhardt 1975) However, the relationship between health and disease seems to be more complex than health being a compass and a trail away from disease. Several incompatible and competing models seem to be at play at the same time: the ideal model, the holistic model, the medical model, and the disjunctive model.

Lastly, and inspired by Engelhardt's seminal work, I argued that there is an increasing gap between disease and diagnosis and between health and its indicators. This has substantial ethical implications for health priority setting and epistemic consequences for disease causality. It also underscores how important philosophical studies of the concepts of health and disease still are 50 years after Engelhard's seminal publication.

References

Album, D., and S. Westin. 2008. Do Diseases Have a Prestige Hierarchy? A Survey Among Physicians and Medical Students. *Social Science & Medicine* 66 (1): 182–188.

Album, D., L. E. Johannessen, and E. B. Rasmussen. 2017. Stability and Change in Disease Prestige: A Comparative Analysis of Three Surveys Spanning a Quarter of a Century. *Social Science & Medicine* 180 (1): 45–51. https://doi.org/10.1016/j.socscimed.2017.03.020.

Ananth, M. 2017. In Defense of an Evolutionary Concept of Health Nature Norms and Human Biology. London: Routledge.

Antonovsky, A. 1985. The life cycle, mental health and the sense of coherence. *The Israel journal of psychiatry and related sciences* 22 (4): 273–80.

Bechtel, William. 1985. In Defense of a Naturalistic Concept of Health. In *Biomedical Ethics Reviews*, ed. James M. Humber and Robert F. Almeder, vol. 1985, 131–170. Humana Press.

Beek, F., P. T. Cohen-Kettenis, and B. P. Kreukels. 2016. Gender Incongruence/Gender Dysphoria and Its Classification History. *International Review of Psychiatry* 28 (1): 5–12. https://doi.org/10.3109/09540261.2015.1091293.

Bickenbach, Jerome. 2015. WHO's Definition of Health: Philosophical Analysis. In *Handbook of the Philosophy of Medicine*, vol. 1.

Bishop, George D., Carole Briede, Laura Cavazos, Roger Grotzinger, and Sharon McMahon. 1987. Processing Illness Information: The Role of Disease Prototypes. *Basic and Applied Social Psychology* 8 (1–2): 21–43.

Boenink, Marianne, and Lennart van der Molen. 2024. The Biomarkerization of Alzheimer's Disease. In *A Pragmatic Approach to Conceptualization of Health and Disease*, ed. Maartje Schermer. Springer Nature.

Bolton, Derek, and Grant Gillett. 2019. *The Biopsychosocial Model of Health and Disease: New Philosophical and Scientific Developments*. Springer Nature.

Boorse, C. 1975. On the Distinction Between Disease and Illness. *Philosophy and Public Affairs* 5:49–68.

Boorse, C. 1977. Health as a Theoretical Concept. *Philosophy of Science* 44:542.

Boorse, C. 2011. Concepts of Health and Disease. In *Philosophy of Medicine*, ed. F. Gifford, 11–34. Burlington; Amsterdam; Oxford: Elsevier.

Boorse, C. 2014. A Second Rebuttal on Health. *The Journal of Medicine and Philosophy* 39 (6): 683–724. https://doi.org/10.1093/jmp/jhu035.

Boyd, K. M. 2000. Disease, Illness, Sickness, Health, Healing and Wholeness: Exploring Some Elusive Concepts. *Medical Humanities* 26:9–17. https://doi.org/10.1136/mh.26.1.9.

Broadbent, A. 2019. Health as a Secondary Property. *The British Journal for the Philosophy of Science* 70 (2): 609–627. https://doi.org/10.1093/bjps/axx014.

Bronfenbrenner, Urie. 1977. Toward an Experimental Ecology of Human Development. *American Psychologist* 32 (7): 513.

Burgess, Alexis, Herman Cappelen, and David Plunkett. 2020. *Conceptual Engineering and Conceptual Ethics*. Oxford University Press.

Burns, Chester R. 1975. Diseases Versus Healths: Some Legacies in the Philosophies of Modern Medical Science. In *Evaluation and Explanation in the Biomedical Sciences*, ed. S. F. Spicker and H. T. Engehlardt, 29–47. Dordrecht: Reidel.

Canguilhem, G. 1989. The Normal and the Pathological. Fawcett CR. Zone Book

Carnap, Rudolf. 1962. On Explication. In *Logical Foundations of Probability*, ed. Rudolf Carnap. Chicago: University of Chicago Press.

Conrad, Peter, and Kristin K. Barker. 2010. The Social Construction of Illness: Key Insights and Policy Implications. *Journal of Health and Social Behavior* 51 (Suppl. 1): S67–S79. https://doi.org/10.1177/0022146510383495. http://hsb.sagepub.com/content/51/1_suppl/S67.abstract.

Cooper, R. 2002. Disease. *Studies in History and Philosophy of Science Part C* 33 (2): 263–282.

Cooper, Rachel. 2017. Health and Disease. In *Bloomsbury Companion to Contemporary Philosophy of Medicine, edited by*, ed. James A. Marcum, 275–296. New York: Bloomsbury Publishing.

De Vreese, Leen. 2017. How to Proceed in the Disease Concept Debate? A Pragmatic Approach. *The Journal of Medicine and Philosophy: A Forum for Bioethics and Philosophy of Medicine* 42 (4): 424–446. https://doi.org/10.1093/jmp/jhx011.

DeVito, S. 2000. On the Value-Neutrality of the Concepts of Health and Disease: Unto the Breach Again. *The Journal of Medicine and Philosophy* 25 (5): 539–567. https://doi.org/10.1076/0360-5310(200010)25:5;1-w;ft539.

Engel, G. L. 1977. The Need for a New Medical Model: A Challenge for Biomedicine. *Science* 196 (4286): 129–136.

Engelhardt, H. T. 1975. The Concepts of Health and Disease. In *Evaluation and Explanation in the Biomedical Sciences*, ed. H. T. Engehlardt and S. F. Spicker, 125–141. Dordrecht: Reidel.

Engelhardt, H. T., and K. W. Wildes. 1995. Health and Disease—Philosophical Perspectives. In *Encyclopedia of Bioethics*, ed. W. T. Reich, 1101–1106. New York: Macmillan.

Ereshefsky, M. 2009. Defining 'Health' and 'Disease'. *Studies in History and Philosophy of Biological and Biomedical Sciences* 40 (3): 221–227. https://doi.org/10.1016/j.shpsc.2009.06.005.

Etches, Vera, John Frank, Erica Di Ruggiero, and Doug Manuel. 2006. Measuring Population Health: A Review of Indicators. *Annual Review of Public Health* 27 (1): 29–55.

Fabrega, H., Jr. 1976. Toward a Theory of Human Disease. *The Journal of Nervous and Mental Disease* 162 (5): 299–312.

Farmer, Paul. 1999. Pathologies of Power: Rethinking Health and Human Rights. *American Journal of Public Health* 89 (10): 1486–1496.

Feinberg, Joel. 1989. *Harm to Self*. Oxford: Oxford University Press.

Gagné-Julien, Anne-Marie. 2024. Beyond Conceptual Analysis: Social Objectivity and Conceptual Engineering to Define Disease. *The Journal of Medicine and Philosophy: A Forum for Bioethics and Philosophy of Medicine* 49 (2): 147–159.

Gangemi, Aldo, Domenico M. Pisanelli, and Geri Steve. 2000. Understanding Systematic Conceptual Structures in Polysemous Medical Terms. In *Proceedings of the AMIA Symposium*. (p. 285).

Gannik, Dorte. 2002. Situational Disease: Elements of a Social Theory of Disease Based on a Study of Back Trouble. *Scandinavian Journal of Primary Health Care* 20 (1): 25–30.

Gerring, John. 1999. What Makes a Concept Good? A Criterial Framework for Understanding Concept Formation in the Social Sciences. *Polity* 31 (3): 357–393.

Gerring, John, Daniel Pemstein, and Svend-Erik Skaaning. 2021. An Ordinal, Concept-Driven Approach to Measurement: The Lexical Scale. *Sociological Methods & Research* 50 (2): 778–811.

Giles, David C. 2014. 'DSM-V Is Taking Away Our identity': The Reaction of the Online Community to the Proposed Changes in the Diagnosis of Asperger's Disorder. *Health* 18 (2): 179–195.

Goosens, William K. 1980. Values, Health, and Medicine. *Philosophy of Science* 47 (1): 100–115.

Griffiths, Paul E., and John Matthewson. 2018. Evolution, Dysfunction, and Disease: A Reappraisal. *The British Journal for the Philosophy of Science* 69 (2): 301–327.

Guerrero, J. David. 2010. On a Naturalist Theory of Health: A Critique. *Studies in History and Philosophy of Science Part C: Studies in History and Philosophy of Biological and Biomedical Sciences* 41 (3): 272–278.

Hacking, I. 1991. *The Social Construction of What?* Cambridge, MA: Harvard University Press.

Hampton, James A. 1995. Testing the Prototype Theory of Concepts. *Journal of Memory and Language* 34 (5): 686–708.

Hampton, J. A. 2007. Typicality, Graded Membership, and Vagueness. *Cognitive Science* 31 (3): 355–384. https://doi.org/10.1080/15326900701326402.

Hare, R. M. 1952. *The Language of Morals*. Oxford: Clarendon Press.

Hare, R. M. 1986. Health. *Journal of Medical Ethics* 12 (4): 174–181.

Hausman, Daniel M. 2012. Health, Naturalism, and Functional Efficiency. *Philosophy of Science* 79 (4): 519–541.

Hausman, D. M. 2014. Health and Functional Efficiency. *The Journal of Medicine and Philosophy* 39 (6): 634–647.

Hauswald, Rico, and Lara Keuck. 2017. Indeterminacy in Medical Classification: On Continuity, Uncertainty, and Vagueness. In *Vagueness in Psychiatry*, ed. G. Keil, L. Keuck, and R. Hauswald, 93–116. Oxford University Press.

Hershenov, David B. 2020. A Naturalist Response to Kingma's Critique of Naturalist Accounts of Disease. *Theoretical Medicine and Bioethics* 41 (2–3): 83–97.

Hesslow, G. 1993. Do We Need a Concept of Disease? *Theoretical Medicine* 14 (1): 1–14.

Hofmann, B. 2001a. Complexity of the Concept of Disease as Shown Through Rival Theoretical Frameworks. *Theoretical Medicine* 22:211–236.

Hofmann, B. 2001b. Complexity of the Concept of Disease as Shown Through Rival Theoretical Frameworks. *Theoretical Medicine and Bioethics* 22 (3): 211–236. http://www.ncbi.nlm.nih.gov/pubmed/11499496.

Hofmann, Bjørn. 2001c. The Technological Invention of Disease. *Medical Humanities* 27 (1): 10–19.

Hofmann, Bjørn. 2005. Simplified Models of the Relationship Between Health and Disease. *Theoretical Medicine and Bioethics* 26 (5): 355–377. https://doi.org/10.1007/s11017-005-7914. Retrieved from http://www.wkap.nl/journalhome.htm/1386-7415.

Hofmann, B. 2010. The Concept of Disease—Vague, Complex, or Just Indefinable? *Medicine, Health Care, and Philosophy* 13 (1): 3–10. https://doi.org/10.1007/s11019-009-9198-7.

Hofmann, Bjørn. 2016. Perspectives on Human Malady: Disease, Illness, and Sickness. In *The Routledge Companion to Philosophy of Medicine*, ed. Miriam Solomon, Jeremy Simon, and Harold Kincaid, 1–11. London: Routledge.

Hofmann, Bjørn. 2017. Technological Invention of Disease. In *Encyclopedia of Creativity, Invention, Innovation and Entrepreneurship*, 1–12. New York, NY: Springer New York.

Hofmann, B. 2018. Looking for Trouble? Diagnostics Expanding Disease and Producing Patients. *Journal of Evaluation in Clinical Practice* 24 (5): 978–982. https://doi.org/10.1111/jep.12941.

Hofmann, Bjørn. 2019a. Human Enhancement: Enhancing Health or Harnessing Happiness? *Journal of Bioethical Inquiry* 16 (1): 87–98.

Hofmann, Bjørn Morten. 2019b. Expanding Disease and Undermining the Ethos of Medicine. *European Journal of Epidemiology (EJE)* 34:613–619. https://doi.org/10.1007/s10654-019-00496-4. https://link.springer.com/journal/10654.

Hofmann, Bjørn. 2021. How to Draw the Line Between Health and Disease? Start with Suffering. *Health Care Analysis* 29 (2): 127–143. https://doi.org/10.1007/s10728-021-00434-0.

Hofmann, Bjørn. 2022a. Acknowledging and Addressing the Many Ethical Aspects of Disease. *Patient Education and Counseling* 105 (5): 1201–1208. https://doi.org/10.1016/j.pec.2021.09.015. https://www.sciencedirect.com/science/article/pii/S0738399121006248.

Hofmann, Bjørn Morten. 2022b. Which Criteria Are (Not) Suitable for Defining the Concept of Disease? *Zeitschrift für medizinische Ethik* 68 (2): 165–178.

Hofmann, Bjørn. 2023a. Addressing the Paradox: Health Expansion Threatening Sustainable Healthcare. *European Journal of Internal Medicine* 117:3–7. https://doi.org/10.1016/j.ejim.2023.09.012. https://www.sciencedirect.com/science/article/pii/S0953620523003321.

Hofmann, Bjørn. 2023b. Does Disease Incite a Stronger Moral Appeal Than Health? *BMC Medicine* 21 (1): 419. https://doi.org/10.1186/s12916-023-03110-3.

Hofmann, Bjørn Morten. 2023c. Aesthetic Injustice. *Journal of Business Ethics* 13. https://doi.org/10.1007/s10551-023-05401-4. http://link.springer.com/journal/10551.

Hofmann, Bjørn. 2024. Moral Obligations Towards Human Persons' Wellbeing Versus Their Suffering: An Analysis of Perspectives of Moral Philosophy. *Health Policy* 142:1–7. https://doi.org/10.1016/j.healthpol.2024.105031

Hofmann, B. M., and H. M. Eriksen. 2001. The Concept of Disease: Ethical Challenges and Relevance to Dentistry and Dental Education. *European Journal of Dental Education* 5 (1): 2–8. discussion 9–11. http://www.ncbi.nlm.nih.gov/pubmed/11168486.

Hofmann, B., and F. Svenaeus. 2018. How Medical Technologies Shape the Experience of Illness. *Life Sciences, Society and Policy* 14 (1): 3. https://doi.org/10.1186/s40504-018-0069-y.

Hofmann, B., K. Bond, and L. Sandman. 2018. Evaluating Facts and Facting Evaluations: On the Fact-Value Relationship in HTA. *Journal of Evaluation in Clinical Practice* 24 (5): 957–965. https://doi.org/10.1111/jep.12920.

Hucklenbroich, Peter. 2017. Disease Entities and the Borderline Between Health and Disease: Where Is the Place of Gradations. In *Vagueness in Psychiatry*, ed. Geert Keil, Lara Keuck, and Rico Hauswald, 75–92. Oxford: Oxford University Press.

Jones, David S., Scott H. Podolsky, and Jeremy A. Greene. 2012. The Burden of Disease and the Changing Task of Medicine. *New England Journal of Medicine* 366 (25): 2333–2338.

Jutel, A., and S. Buetow. 2007. A Picture of Health? Unmasking the Role of Appearance in Health. *Perspectives in Biology and Medicine* 50 (3): 421–434. https://doi.org/10.1353/pbm.2007.0032.

Kaebnick, Gregory E. 2013. *Humans in Nature: The World as We Find It and the World as We Create It*. Oxford: Oxford University Press.

Keil, Geert, and Ralf Stoecker. 2016. *Disease as a Vague and Thick Cluster Concept*. Vagueness in Psychiatry.

Kendler, Kenneth S. 2010. The Rise and Fall of the Biopsychosocial Model: Reconciling Art and Science in Psychiatry. *American Journal of Psychiatry* 167 (8): 999–1000. https://doi.org/10.1176/appi.ajp.2010.10020268.

Khushf, G. 2007. An Agenda for Future Debate on Concepts of Health and Disease. *Medicine, Health Care, and Philosophy* 10 (1): 19–27.; discussion 29–32. https://doi.org/10.1007/s11019-006-9021-7.

King, L. 1954. What is a Disease? *Philosophy of Science* 21 (3): 193–203.

Kingma, E. 2014. Naturalism About Health and Disease: Adding Nuance for Progress. *The Journal of Medicine and Philosophy* 39 (6): 590–608. https://doi.org/10.1093/jmp/jhu037.

Kingma, Elselijn. 2017. Disease as Scientific and as Value-Laden Concept. *Handbook of the Philosophy of Medicine* 1:45–63.

Kingsbury, Justine, and Jonathan McKeown-Green. 2009. Definitions: Does Disjunction Mean Dysfunction? *The Journal of Philosophy* 106 (10): 568–585.

Knobe, Joshua, Sandeep Prasada, and George E. Newman. 2013. Dual Character Concepts and the Normative Dimension of Conceptual Representation. *Cognition* 127 (2): 242–257.

Kovacs, J. 1998. The Concept of Health and Disease. *Medicine, Health Care, and Philosophy* 1 (1): 31–39.

Kukla, Rebecca. 2014. Medicalization,"Normal Function," and the Definition of Health. In *The Routledge Companion to Bioethics*, 539–554. Routledge.

Lakoff, George, and Mark Johnson. 1999. *Philosophy in the Flesh: The Embodied Mind and Its Challenge to Western Thought*. Basic Books.

Lalljee, Mansur, Roger Lamb, and Giovanni Carnibella. 1993. Lay Prototypes of Illness: Their Content and Use. *Psychology and Health* 8 (1): 33–49.

Levin, Jeff, and Matt Bradshaw. 2023. Normal Isn't Normal: On the Medicalization of Health. *EXPLORE* 20 (3): 417–423. https://doi.org/10.1016/j.explore.2023.10.008.

Lindstrøm, Jon A. 2012. Medico-Ethical Versus Biological Evaluationism, and the Concept of Disease. *Medicine, Health Care and Philosophy* 15 (2): 165–173.

Martin, Mike W. 2006. *From Morality to Mental Health: Virtue and Vice in a Therapeutic Culture*. Oxford University Press.

Martin, C. M., and C. Peterson. 2009. The Social Construction of Chronicity—A Key to Understanding Chronic Care Transformations. *Journal of Evaluation in Clinical Practice* 15 (3): 578–585. https://doi.org/10.1111/j.1365-2753.2008.01025.x.

Matthewson, John, and Paul E. Griffiths. 2017. Biological Criteria of Disease: Four Ways of Going Wrong. *The Journal of Medicine and Philosophy: A Forum for Bioethics and Philosophy of Medicine* 42 (4): 447–466. https://doi.org/10.1093/jmp/jhx004.

Metzler, Ingrid. 2010. Biomarkers and Their Consequences for the Biomedical Profession: A Social Science Perspective. *Personalized Medicine* 7 (4): 407–420.

Nordenfelt, L. 1986. Health and Disease: Two Philosophical Perspectives. *Journal of Epidemiology and Community Health* 40 (4): 281–284.

Nordenfelt, L. 1993. On the Relevance and Importance of the Notion of Disease. *Theoretical Medicine* 14 (1): 15–26.

Nordenfelt, Lennart. 1995. On the Ontology of Disease. In *On the Nature of Health: An Action-Theoretic Approach*, 151–173. Dordrecht: Springer Netherlands.

Nordenfelt, L. 2000. On the Place of Fuzzy Health in Medical Theory. *The Journal of Medicine and Philosophy* 25 (5): 639–649. https://doi.org/10.1076/0360-5310(200010)25:5;1-w;ft639.

Nordenfelt, L. 2005. *On the Nature of Health*. Dordrecht: Kluwer Academic Publishers.

Nordenfelt, L. 2007. The Concepts of Health and Illness Revisited. *Medicine, Health Care, and Philosophy* 10 (1): 5–10. https://doi.org/10.1007/s11019-006-9017-3.

Nordenfelt, L. 2013. The Opposition Between Naturalistic and Holistic Theories of Health and Disease. In *Health, Illness and Disease: Philosophical Essays*, ed. H. Carel and R. Cooper. London, New York: Routledge.

Osler, William. 1916. *The Principles and Practice of Medicine*. New York: D. Appleton and Company.

Papa, Frank J., and Feiming Li. 2015. Evidence of the Preferential Use of Disease Prototypes Over Case Exemplars Among Early Year One Medical Students Prior to and Following Diagnostic Training. *Diagnosis* 2 (4): 217–225.

Paul, Farmer. 2003. Pathologies of Power. In *Health, Human Rights and the New War on the Poor*. Berkeley: University of California Press.

Pörn, I. 1984. An equilibrium model of health. In: Nordenfelt L, Linddahl B, eds. Health, disease, and causal explanations in medicine. *Reidel Publishing Company* 3–9.

Pörn, I. 1993. Health and adaptedness. *Theoretical medicine* 14 (4): 295–303.

Powell, Russell, and Eric Scarffe. 2019. Rethinking "Disease": A Fresh Diagnosis and a New philoSophical Treatment. *Journal of Medical Ethics* 45 (9): 579–588. https://doi.org/10.1136/medethics-2019-105465. https://jme.bmj.com/content/medethics/45/9/579.full.pdf.

Recio, D. M. A. 1974. A united concept of health and illness. ANPHI Pap. Jan-Jun9(1-2): 22–6.

Reznek, L. 1987. *The Nature of Disease*. New York: Routledge & Keagen Paul.

Richardson, Henry S. 2016. Capabilities and the Definition of Health: Comments on Venkatapuram. *Bioethics* 30 (1): 1–7.

Rogers, W. A., and M. J. Walker. 2017. The Line-Drawing Problem in Disease Definition. *The Journal of Medicine and Philosophy* 42 (4): 405–423. https://doi.org/10.1093/jmp/jhx010.

Rogers, W. A., and M. J. Walker. 2018. Précising Definitions as a Way to Combat Overdiagnosis. *Journal of Evaluation in Clinical Practice* 24 (5): 1019–1025.

Rose, Nikolas. 2009. *The Politics of Life Itself: Biomedicine, Power, and Subjectivity in the Twenty-First Century*. Princeton NJ: Princeton University Press.

Sade, R. M. 1995. A Theory of Health and Disease: The Objectivist-Subjectivist Dichotomy. *The Journal of Medicine and Philosophy* 20 (5): 513–525.

Sadegh-Zadeh, K. 2000. Fuzzy Health, Illness, and Disease. *The Journal of Medicine and Philosophy* 25 (5): 605–638. https://doi.org/10.1076/0360-5310(200010)25:5;1-w;ft605.

Sadegh-Zadeh, K. 2008. The Prototype Resemblance Theory of Disease. *The Journal of Medicine and Philosophy* 33 (2): 106–139. https://doi.org/10.1093/jmp/jhn004.

Schroeder, S. Andrew. 2013. Rethinking Health: Healthy or Healthier Than? *The British Journal for the Philosophy of Science* 64 (1): 131–159. https://doi.org/10.1093/bjps/axs006. http://bjps.oxfordjournals.org/content/64/1/131.abstract.

Sedgwick, P. 1973. Illness--Mental and Otherwise. *Hastings Center Studies* 1 (3): 19–40.

Seising, R. 2006. From Vagueness in Medical Thought to the Foundations of Fuzzy Reasoning in Medical Diagnosis. *Artificial Intelligence in Medicine* 38 (3): 237–256. https://doi.org/10.1016/j.artmed.2006.06.004.

Sharf, B. F., and M. L. Vanderford. 2003. Illness narratives and the social construction of health. *The Routledge handbook of health communication*, 23–48. Routledge.

Sholl, Jonathan, and Simon Okholm. 2021. Taking a Naturalistic Turn in the Health and Disease Debate. *Teorema: Revista Internacional de Filosofia* 40 (1): 91–110.

Sigerist, Henry E. 1941. The Value of Health to a City. Two Lectures, Delivered in 1873, by MAX VON PETTENKOFER, Translated from the German, with an Introduction. *Bulletin of the History of Medicine* 10: 473.

Sim, Daniel, Michael C. Brothers, Joseph M. Slocik, Ahmad E. Islam, Benji Maruyama, Claude C. Grigsby, Rajesh R. Naik, and Steve S. Kim. 2022. Biomarkers and Detection Platforms for Human Health and Performance Monitoring: A Review. *Advanced Science* 9 (7): 2104426.

Stempsey, William E. 1999. *Disease and Diagnosis: Value-Dependant Realism*. Dortrecht: Kluwer.

Stoecker, Ralf, and Geert Keil. 2016. Disease as a Vague and Thick Cluster Concept. In *Vagueness in Psychiatry*, ed. Geert Keil, Lara Keuck, and Rico Hauswald, 46–74. Oxford: Oxford University Press.

Szasz, Thomas S. 1960. The Myth of Mental Illness. *American Psychologist* 15 (2): 113.

Tristram Engelhardt, H., Jr. 1973. Psychotherapy as Meta-Ethics. *Psychiatry* 36 (4): 440–445.

van der Linden, Rik, and Maartje Schermer. 2022. Health and Disease as Practical Concepts: Exploring Function in Context-Specific Definitions. *Medicine, Health Care and Philosophy* 25 (1): 131–140. https://doi.org/10.1007/s11019-021-10058-9.

Vandamme, D., W. Fitzmaurice, B. Kholodenko, and W. Kolch. 2013. Systems Medicine: Helping Us Understand the Complexity of Disease. *QJM: An International Journal of Medicine* 106 (10): 891–895.

VanderWeele, Tyler J., Eileen McNeely, and Howard K. Koh. 2019. Reimagining Health—Flourishing. *JAMA* 321 (17): 1667–1668. https://doi.org/10.1001/jama.2019.3035

Veit, Walter. 2021. Biological Normativity: A New Hope for Naturalism? *Medicine, Health Care and Philosophy* 24 (2): 291–301. https://doi.org/10.1007/s11019-020-09993-w.

Venkatapuram, Sridhar. 2009. *Health and Justice: The Capability to be Healthy*. University of Cambridge.

Venkatapuram, S. 2013. Health, vital goals, and central human capabilities. *Bioethics* 27 (5): 271–279. https://doi.org/10.1111/j.1467-8519.2011.01953.x

Visser, Alnica. 2023. *In Defense of Concept Variability*. University of Pittsburgh.

Vogt, Henrik, and Bjørn Morten Hofmann. 2022. How Precision Medicine Changes Medical Epistemology: A Formative Case from Norway. *Journal of Evaluation in Clinical Practice* 28 (6): 1205–1212. https://doi.org/10.1111/jep.13649. http://www.blackwellpublishing.com/journal.asp?ref=1356-1294&site=1.

Wakefield, J. C. 1999. Evolutionary Versus Prototype Analyses of the Concept of Disorder. *Journal of Abnormal Psychology* 108 (3): 374–399.

Wakefield, J. C. 2007. The Concept of Mental Disorder: Diagnostic Implications of the Harmful Dysfunction Analysis. *World Psychiatry* 6 (3): 149–156.

Wakefield, J. C. 2013. DSM-5 Grief Scorecard: Assessment and Outcomes of Proposals to Pathologize Grief. *World Psychiatry* 12 (2): 171–173. https://doi.org/10.1002/wps.20053.

Wakefield, J. C. 2014. The Biostatistical Theory Versus the Harmful Dysfunction Analysis, Part 1: Is Part-Dysfunction a Sufficient Condition for Medical Disorder? *The Journal of Medicine and Philosophy* 39 (6): 648–682. https://doi.org/10.1093/jmp/jhu038.

Walker, Mary Jean, and Wendy A. Rogers. 2018. A New Approach to Defining Disease. *The Journal of Medicine and Philosophy: A Forum for Bioethics and Philosophy of Medicine* 43 (4): 402–420. https://doi.org/10.1093/jmp/jhy014.

Whitbeck, Caroline. 1977. Causation in Medicine: The Disease Entity Model. *Philosophy of Science* 44 (4): 619–637.

Whitbeck, C. 1981. A Theory of Health. In *Concepts of Health and Disease: Interdisciplinary Perspectives*, ed. H. T. Engelhardt, A. L. Caplan, and J. J. McCartney. Reading, Mass: Addison-Wesley.

Wieland, Wolfgang. 2013. Diagnose. In *Diagnose*. de Gruyter.

Wittgenstein, Ludwig. 1958. *The Blue and Brown Books*. Vol. 18. Oxford: Blackwell Oxford.

World Health Organization. 1946. Preamble to the Constitution of the World Health Organization.

Worrall, Jennifer, and John Worrall. 2001. Defining Disease: Much Ado About Nothing? In *Life Interpretation and the Sense of Illness Within the Human Condition*, Analecta Husserliana, ed. Anna-Teresa Tymieniecka and Evandro Agazzi, 33–55. Springer Netherlands.

Chapter 3
The Concepts of Health and Disease

H. Tristram Engelhardt Jr

Health and disease are cardinal concepts of the biomedical sciences and technologies. Though the models of health and disease may vary, these concepts play a defining role, indicating what should and what should not be the objects of medical concern. The concepts are ambiguous, operating both as explanatory and evaluatory notions. They describe states of affairs, factual conditions, while at the same time judging them to be good or bad. Health and disease are normative as well as descriptive. This dual role is core to their ambiguity and is the focus of this paper. In this paper I shall examine first the concept of health; second, the concept of disease; and third, I will draw some general conclusions concerning the interplay of evaluation and explanation in the concepts of health and disease.

3.1 Health

Health is a normative concept but not in the sense of a moral virtue. Though health is a good, and though it may be morally praiseworthy to try to be healthy and to advance the health of others, still, all things being equal, it is a misfortune, not a misdeed, to lack health. Health is more an aesthetic than an ethical term; it is more

This chapter originally appeared as H. Tristram Engelhardt, Jr., "The Concepts of Health and Disease," in *Evaluation and Explanation in the Biomedical Sciences*, ed. H.T. Engehlardt, Jr. and S.F. Spicker (Reidel), 125–141. Reprinted with permission from Springer.

H. Tristram Engelhardt Jr died before publication of this work was completed.

H. Tristram Engelhardt Jr (✉)
Galveston, TX, USA

L. M. Rasmussen, S. Holm (eds.), *50 Years of Philosophy and Medicine*,
Philosophy and Medicine 150, https://doi.org/10.1007/978-3-031-95175-6_3

beauty than virtue. Thus, one does not condemn someone for no longer being healthy, though one may sympathize with him over the loss of a good Further, it is not clear exactly what is lost when one loses health.

The norms of health are difficult to compass within one homogeneous concept, in particular within an independent definition which does not define health negatively, as the absence of disease. The World Health Organization attempted a positive definition, that "health is a state of complete physical, mental and social well-being and not merely the absence of disease or infirmity" (Constitution of the World Health Organization 1958). But such a definition of health packs the ambiguity of the concept of health into the ambiguity of a concept of well-being. Further, this concept of well-being suggests the notion of a satisfactory lifestyle, including successful adaptation to one's environment Yet, even here the norms are obscure. What is a good adaptation? Is a good adaptation possible in a complex industrial society for those with I.Q.'s of less than 80? Are such persons ill? Further, if health is a state of complete physical, mental and social well-being, can anyone ever be healthy? Does health become a regulative ideal, one to which one strives, but which one can never fully achieve? On the other hand, if no one is truly healthy, is everyone ill? Are health and disease exclusive or overlapping concepts?

These quandaries arise primarily out of the evaluatory, not the explanatory, dimension of the concepts of health and disease. Health could, for example, be defined as the ability to perform those functions which allow the organism to maintain itself, all other things being equal, in the range of activity open to most other members of its species (e.g., within two standard deviations from the norm), and which are conducive toward the maintenance of its species. This, though, is to forego mention of why one might be interested in certain types of well-being (except for the commitment to the survival of the species). Also, it is not clear whether, within such a concept, degenerative processes generally distributed in the population, which appear after the reproductive years, could count as diseases. Finally, if health is to encompass issues raised by particular diseases, the concept may lose its unity. The attempt to understand the concept of health thus brings us to the concept of disease, suggesting that the concept of health may have as many nuances as there are diseases, and that it may be derivative from these particular disease concepts.

3.2 The Concept of Disease

The concept of disease is used in accounting for physiological and psychological (or behavioral) disorders, offering generalizations concerning patterns of phenomena which we find disturbing and unpleasant. The concept of disease is a general scheme for explaining, predicting, and controlling dimensions of the human condition. It grades into other concepts which are political, social, educational, and moral. The difference between the concept of disease and these other concepts, and the similarity of the various models of disease is complex and problematic. It is not even clear that all the models of disease fall within a single genus. Perhaps the concept of disease indicates a family of conceptually consanguineous notions. That is, the concept of disease may be a basically heterogeneous concept standing for a set of phenomena collected together out of diverse social interests, not on the basis of the recognition of a natural type or a common conceptual structure. Disease would then be whatever physicians in a particular society treat, rendering circular the definitions of disease and medicine.

It is worthwhile distinguishing, somewhat stipulatively, disease and illness. One can be ill, feel bad, feel under the weather without explaining such phenomena in terms of disease models. The concept of disease competes with other concepts, from demonic possession to simple exhaustion. And, on the other hand, one can have a disease without being ill, as in the case of Alvan Feinstein's concept of lanthanic diseases (Feinstein 1967). A person can, for example, have carcinoma of the lung diagnosed before he is ill. To speak of diseases is to make an explanatory move and at the very least to convert an illness into a syndrome, to recognize a cluster of phenomena as a disease pattern.

The concept of disease acts not only to describe and explain, but also to enjoin to action. It indicates a state of affairs as undesirable and to be overcome. It is a normative concept; it says what ought not to be. As such, the concept incorporates criteria of evaluation, designating certain states of affairs as desirable and others as not so. It delineates and establishes social roles such as being sick or being a physician, and it interconnects these roles with a network of expectations structured by rights and duties (Siegler and Osmond 1973). The concept is both aesthetic and ethical, suggesting what is beautiful and what is good. By terming something diseased, one indicates that the state of affairs is both naturally ugly as well as one that imposes some obligations and relieves others.

The concept of disease is thus freighted with important ambiguities. These ambiguities are, as well, bound to what has been termed the physiological and ontological concepts of disease, to the levels of abstraction involved in disease models, and to the nature of particular models of disease, such as the medical and psychological. I wish to introduce the physiological and ontological concepts of disease from a primarily typological, not historical, point of view. They represent two general ways of talking about disease. Historically, they developed out of disputes whether disease was the result of the malmixing of humors, or was due to the entrance of a disease entity. The dispute roughly was whether diseases were primarily relational and contextual in character, or in some sense substantial things. These different ways of talking about disease are still apparent.

There is an important ambiguity in the significance of ontological concepts of disease. The *ens*, the being of the disease, can be variously understood as either a thing, or a logical type, or both. Medical ontology in the strong sense refers to views in which disease is conceived of as a thing, a parasite (Engelhardt 1974a), in contrast with "Platonic" views of disease entities in which diseases are understood as unchanging conceptual structures. In the strong sense a "disease entity" is a disease thing, a material, invading agent of disease (Sigerist 1932, 105–106). This strong sense of ontology involves a commitment to hypostatization, an attempt to reify disease. For example, Paracelsus, whom Pagel describes as the prototypical ontologist, opposed the humoral pathologists who held that "the sick individual determines the cause and nature of disease." In contrast, Paracelsus taught "the 'ontological' view in which diseases are regarded as entities in themselves distinguishable by specific changes and causes." In this view, it was "the individual disease that conditions the patient and manifests itself in a characteristic picture" (Pagel 1958). This analysis suggested that specific therapies should be sought for specific diseases. Or, more fundamentally, it advanced the notion that diseases had specific characters, and would thus respond to specific therapies. Moreover, his view suggested a distinction between "symptomatic" and "aetiological" therapy, therapy aimed at the results and therapy aimed at the cause of disease. It was this ontological, aetiological concept of disease which indicated the possibility of classifying therapies according to their focus on the specific causes of diseases. Further, specific diseases led to specific local organ changes being sought by van Helmont and others, and thus to the beginning of modern pathology (Pagel 1944). The identification of disease with particular causes, therapies, and, finally, with localized pathological changes in organs is the focus of this viewpoint.

The ontological concept of disease spans the meaning of disease from Paracelsus' concept of the disease as a parasite, to concepts of contagion as found in Harvey (Pagel and Winder 1968), to modern bacteriological concepts in which illness is variously identified with infectious agents. Bacteriology finally vindicated Sydenham's faith in the possibility of specific remedies for specific diseases. As Knud Faber put it, diseases "came to be viewed from an etiological point of view, and the efforts of clinicians were directed towards… a nosography founded on the morbific causes" (Faber 1923, 98; see also 108–109). The picture emerged of the host, the environment, and the disease agent as the elements of disease with the accent falling heavily on the agent of disease, particularly as an infectious agent. As Rudolf Virchow remarked, this "idea of particular, parasitic disease entities is without doubt ontological in an outspoken manner" (Virchow 1895). This ontological view involves as well a confusion of the cause of illness and the disease itself, as when the disease, tuberculosis, is identified with Mycobacterium tuberculosis. Virchow saw this as beginning with the discovery of microorganisms and presupposing a "hopeless, never-ending confusion, in which the ideas of being (*ens morbi*) and causation (*causa morbi*) have been arbitrarily thrown together" (Virchow 1895). In this, Virchow was undoubtedly correct. He, though, was himself also, by his own admission, "a thoroughgoing ontologist," who identified the pathological findings as the *ens morbi*, the disease entity (Virchow 1895). Though he eschewed one form of reifying nosology, he embraced another. Disease became specific pathological changes in specific cells.

But the move to reification is only one dimension of the ontological thesis concerning disease. The other dimension is bound to a judgment concerning the nature of the disease pattern, the constellation or cluster of the signs and symptoms which form the character of a disease. In ontological theories, these characteristic disease patterns are interpreted as enduring disease types often without an immediate connection to a particular theory of material disease entities. It is an ontological question (in the philosophical sense) of the reality of disease types, one that asserts that they have a being beyond their particular instantiations. This interpretation of illnesses as portraying natural or essential disease types suggests an almost Platonic construal. In this view, courses of illnesses more or less fully achieve a natural type. Classical cases of a disease are thus perfect instantiations of a disease type and atypical cases imperfect realizations of a disease reality which exists as a natural, logical possibility. "Ontological" in this sense refers to claims of a reality for diseases existing apart from their embodiment in actual illnesses, which illnesses may be "atypical."

It is not clear that anyone held a fully realist view of diseases, but it is a viewpoint presupposed in the ordinary discussions of hospital wards where reference is made to "cases of *X* disease" in a way parallel with phrases such as "instances of *X* idea." To talk of illnesses achieving certain constant and real patterns, best illustrated by classical cases, and obscured by atypical cases, is to talk in a realist mode. To a point, it is illustrated by such classical nosologies as that of Francois Boissier de Sauvages (1706–1767), *Nosologia Methodica* (de Sauvages 1768). Even with his empirical dedication, symptom constellations were for Sauvages types of diseases. Pinel's *Nosographie philosophique* (Pinel 1798). distinguished the varying symptoms of diseases from the "essential fevers," and attracted Broussais' classical critique of ontological theories of diseases. "One has filled the nosographical framework with groups of most arbitrarily formed symptoms… which do not represent the affections of different organs, that is, the real diseases. These groups of symptoms are derived from entities or abstract beings, which are most completely artificial ονtοι; these entities are false, and the resulting treatise is ontological" (Broussais 1821). As Peter Niebyl indicated, Broussais' objection was against abstraction, not against the specificity of disease entities (1971, 118). The moral of the story is that there are strong Platonic, realist tendencies in talk about diseases, and that the tendencies have met opposition from anti-realist quarters bearing a resemblance, if only distant, to the old humoral theories. When viewed in contrast to such anti-realist theories, ontological theories of disease indicate more "the ever-recurring craving of… clinicians for… fixed categories of diseases," (Faber 1923), than an attempt to reify disease concepts, which I have called medical ontology in the strong sense. The ontological sense of disease thus spans a range of significance from the concept of a specific logical entity to a specific material entity.

The traditional viewpoint contrasting with that of the ontologist has been the physiological or functional viewpoint Lord Cohen drew the contrast as between a Platonic, realist, rationalist versus a Hippocratic, nominalistic, empirical view of disease (Cohen 1960, 160). The argument against ontological concepts was, as Wunderlich realized, an argument against the logical blunder of confusing abstract concepts with things, "presupposing them as actually existing and at once considering and treating them as entities," as well as against "models of diseases which contain no truly essential feature… [and] to which we only by way of exception or by using compulsion, find an example in nature" (Wunderlich 1842). But it was not a denial that there are patterns of disease processes. Essential disease types are not the same as basic laws of physiology or pathophysiology.

Those arguing for a physiological concept of disease had at least three points to make, which individual nosologists made more or less completely. First, they wished to secure the concept of disease as a general, not a specific notion. That is, they wished to make diseases functions of the general laws of physiology rather than functions of the more particular laws of the pathology of specific diseases. Yet, second, they wished to argue for a greater appreciation of the individuality of illnesses so that every particular disease-state could be understood in terms of its particular departures from general physiological norms. Heinrich Romberg put it this way, "And we do not regard the mere placing of the disease under this or that rubric as the final aim of diagnosis.... The most important thing remains the determination of the degree that the individual human is injured by his malady, and which cause has produced the momentary disorder" (Romberg 1909, 4). Third, they wished to avoid the metaphysical and logical muddles of ontological concepts of disease. Diseases were not things nor were they perduring types of pathology. Rather, for the physiological or functional nosologists, diseases were more contextual than substantial, more the resultant of individual constitutions, the laws of physiology and the peculiarities of environment, than the result of disease entities. The physiological nosologists were closer to the Hippocratic appreciation of the nexus of airs, waters, and places.

The dispute between ontological and physiological theories of disease turns centrally on the ontological and logical status of disease entities. Ontological theorists framed views within which diseases could be appreciated as specific entities. Physiological theorists framed views within which diseases could be appreciated as particular deviations from general regularities. In the first case, the accent of reality fell upon the disease; in the second case the accent fell upon the individual and his circumstances, including the laws of physiology. There is a temptation to see this contrast as between a realist and a nominalist construal of the meaning of disease. There are surely strongly nominalist leitmotifs in physiological and functional theories of disease. There is an emphasis upon the individual, not the disease, as the reality in the illness. But though there is a sympathy with nominalism, there is no commitment; physiological theorists have been willing to speak of diseases and accord them a conceptual reality. For example, Ottomar Rosenbach's term, "ventricular insufficiency," indicated a disease state which has a real universality, though no reality apart from the instances of which it is the common property. It is a similarity between processes but not a thing, nor a disease entity with a unique cause. It is a resemblance common to a family of processes, not just a family of processes collected together out of various resemblances.

In the end it is because of the need for universality that both ontological and physiological disease theorists required more than a nominalism, though less than a full-blown realism. Progress from syndromes to disease entities helped secure the possibility of diagnosis, prognosis, and therapy, or, more generally, medicine's explanation, prediction, and control of reality. More than the mere ability to name similar objects, one needed as well to indicate a common structure in reality, even if that structure was only the physiological norms from which diseases were departures. Mere syndromes are, as the name implies, the running together of symptoms and signs. They are a constellation of phenomena without a nomological structure to bind the signs and symptoms in a fashion to provide a model for explanation. Treatment and prognosis concerning mere syndromes are empiric in the derogatory sense of a maneuver based on correlations but devoid of an account of the relation between the phenomena correlated. Disease entities offered a level of abstraction that could bind together the signs and symptoms in an etiological matrix. In particular, reifying medical ontological theories could treat diseases as the substances which bear the signs and symptoms, the accidents of the underlying essential reality. Thus identification of phthisis with Mycobacterium tuberculosis or with anatomical pathological findings gave a picture in terms of which the phenomena associated with the clinical entity, consumption, could be collected and organized. This organization involved the binding of the phenomena of the syndrome to the etiological matrix of pathophysiological laws. The temptation was, though, as has been illustrated, to reify the matrix as an *ens morbi* – to, as Virchow remarked, treat disease as "a real substance (*ens*)" (Virchow 1895).

Similarly, the realist ontological theories involved a commitment to disease types. But reality was closer to that of the physiological theorists in being etiologically open – disease entities did not prove to have unique etiologies. As Virchow indicated, known pathogens can exist in hosts without pathology (Virchow 1895). Disease causality is equivocal. Diseases are, as the physiological nosologists stressed, much more complex than the easy simplicity implicit in many ontological nosologies. Diseases are, in fact, not only multifactorial, but multidimensional, involving genetic, physiological, psychological, and sociological components. The presence of these various components does not merely entail a superimposition of modifying variables upon basic disease structures. Rather, it implies that diseases have a basically relational, not a subject (i.e., substance)-predicate (accident) nature. That is, there is not necessarily a *bearer* for every disease, a substrate for each type of disease.

This view of disease emerges from consideration of the complex of etiological structures involved in modern "disease entities." Diseases such as asthma, cancer, coronary artery disease, etc., are as much psychological as pathophysiological in that the likelihood of such illness is closely bound to experienced stress and the availability of support for the person stressed (Holmes and Rahe 1967). They are thus sociological as well. The result is a multidimensional concept of disease with each dimension – genetic, infectious, metabolic, psychological and social – containing a nexus of causes bound by their appropriate, usually different, nomological structures. The multiple factors in such well-established diseases as coronary artery disease suggest that the disease could be alternatively construed as a genetic, metabolic, anatomic, psychological, or sociological disease, depending on whether one was a geneticist, an internist, a surgeon, a psychiatrist, or a public health official. The construal would depend upon the particular scientist's appraisal of which etiological variables were most amenable to his manipulations. For example, the public health official may decide that the basic variables in coronary artery disease are elements of a lifestyle which includes little exercise, overeating and cigarette smoking. He may then address these social variables and consider such diseases to be, as Stewart Wolf suggested, ways of life (Wolf 1961).

This shift in nosology is back to a "Hippocratic" notion of disease in the sense of a "physiological" or contextual concept. The Greeks have been criticized for producing "many separate disease entities, but never [arriving] at the concept of specific etiology" (Hudson 1966). In a sense, the criticism is justified. The Greeks described syndromes, but did not succeed in providing nomological substructures for diseases so that reliable explanation, prediction, and control of reality (i.e., diagnosis, prognosis, and therapy) were possible. The ontological nosologies can somewhat summarily be described as a response to this shortcoming; they were a move to a further level of abstraction allowing the signs and symptoms clustered in a disease to be understood as the appearance of either a disease-thing (an *ens morbi*), or a specific disease pattern. But the actual complexity of diseases suggests that though Hippocratic medicine failed to advance successfully a general account of the syndromes it described, it was properly cautious in not accepting theories of specific etiologies.

Conclusions in this area are at best tentative. But the ever more frequent epidemiological studies of disease, such as the Framingham study of cardiovascular disease, indicate a pattern-pattern analysis within which the pattern of signs and symptoms clustering in a syndrome is bound to a pattern of causal variables (U.S. National Heart Institute 1968). Appearance is bound to a nomological substructure, with both levels having a fairly open-ended character. Moreover, this open-endedness is controlled by pragmatic interests which can bring the disease to a genetic, metabolic, psychological, or social focus, etc., depending on which variables are to be manipulated. Such focusing, though, does not require a reduction of other variables. That is, the genetic variables in heart disease are not reduced to occult sociological variables when one focuses on the elements of lifestyle central to treating heart disease. They are rather treated as mediate variables placed in relation to a model which has sociological variables and correlations as its central structure. One abandons ontological hypostatization of disease and nosological realism, and construes the reality of disease as a conceptual nexus posited for understanding the world of appearance.

Where does this put us with regard to models of disease? The adoption of either a medical or psychological model is a pragmatic choice to focus on a particular cluster of variables and their correlations in order to make certain explanatory, predictive, and controlling maneuvers. But, to isolate these distinguishable dimensions of diseases, is to separate that which is distinguishable but of one fabric. The question of the correct model is either a pragmatic question or a misunderstanding. All diseases can be construed as both medical and psychological; only a confirmed Cartesian would hold that the models are totally separable, while only a monist would hold that they are not distinguishable. To assert that there is not a somatic substrate for psychological events is to assert that psychological life takes place nowhere in this world, that it is the enterprise of an at least partially nonembodied spirit. If human experience and action is to be integrated in and for this world, it must occur somewhere in this world. On the other hand, those psychological generalizations which coordinate mental events in terms of drives and inclinations are distinguishable as such from models free of such intentional predicates and generalizations (Engelhardt 1973a). If mind and body are not two substances but two distinguishable levels of human significance, concerning which generalizations of different characters can be made, as indeed does appear to be the case, then medical and psychological models of disease should be complementary, not competitive. They should complete what would otherwise be one-sided assertions concerning a particular model.

The concept of disease is an attempt to correlate constellations of signs and symptoms for the purposes of explanation, prediction, and control. Pitfalls exist, such as the temptation to reify diseases or to treat. diseases as rigid, specific types with unique etiologies. Diseases involve patterns of causes correlated with clusters of signs and symptoms which constitute the illnesses at hand. Disease models, as nomological patterns, are interpretable in larger patterns in a way not readily apparent if those models modeled disease things or independent disease types. Thus, one can concomitantly have a medical and a psychological account of the etiology of coronary artery disease, which are not incompatible, but mutually completing. That is, the models are not modeling two different things, nor are they two models of the same thing – a disease thing. Rather, they are two modes of correlating variables intrinsic and extrinsic to an ill person. The variables are chosen for the purpose of speaking about and altering that illness. They are relationships structured for particular diagnostic, prognostic, and therapeutic goals, and are based on distinctions between psychological and physical phenomena, between psychological and physical predicates. The issue of the medical versus the psychological model of disease is thus a rehearsal of the mind-body problem. It is bound in part to the claim that diseases are things, with the consequent problem whether a disease thing can have a psychological reality. The identification of objectivity with physical descriptions suggests that if diseases are things, then they have nothing to do with the subjective world of values and social relations often imported into concepts of mental illness. Under such a view, mental illnesses could be diseases only if they described the malfunctioning of a mental thing (e.g., a *res cogitans*).

Criticisms of medical model accounts of mental illness are heterogeneous (Macklin 1972). The critique given by Szasz turns in part on the notion that problems in living are diseases only if they have a physical basis and that, moreover, true diseases are value-free (Szasz 1960). Under this view, all diseases are medical diseases. As a consequence, in such a view psychiatry becomes a moral enterprise where blame and praise (i.e., responsibility for one's own actions) are more appropriate than treatment, prognosis, and therapy (Szasz 1965). The myth of mental illness is the myth that the autonomy of mental life is intrinsically undermined by disease. Disease in this account is identical with a form of reductionism which hides social judgment under claims to scientific objectivity. The assumption is that medicine deals with things and that psychology deals with broader issues such as social development (Albee 1969). But if diseases are means for coordinating phenomena for the purposes of prognosis, diagnosis, and therapy, then the issues can be reformulated not only to allow for the coordination of mental phenomena in diseases, but for the intrusion of values into medical models of diseases as well. To talk of diseases, and an intrinsic role for values in medical diseases, is to abandon ontological nosological analyses of disease and replace them with a contextual view closer to the more open-ended physiological nosologies of the past.

Diseases such as cancer, tuberculosis, and schizophrenia thus exist, but as patterns of explanation, not as things in themselves or as eidetic types of phenomena. Owsei Temkin comes close to such an appreciation of the plastic nature of the concept of disease. "The question: does disease exist or are there only sick persons? is an abstract one and, in that form, does not allow a meaningful answer. Disease is not simply either the one or the other. Rather, it must be thought of as the circumstance requires. The circumstances are represented by the patient, the physician, the public health man, the medical scientist, the pharmaceutical industry, society at large, and last but not least, the disease itself" (Temkin 1961). But the disease in itself is in the end the disease as it exists for us who both experience illness and explain it. Disease as an explanatory account is bound to the circumstances of that account. In short, explanatory accounts are not things; things are what explanatory accounts explain and disease is a mode for explaining things – in particular, ill humans.

The portrayal of particular diseases involves pragmatic judgments which ontological nosologies reified or stereotyped. C. S. Peirce argued that "*In order to ascertain the meaning of an intellectual conception one should consider what practical consequences might conceivably result by necessity from the truth of that conception; and the sum of these consequences will constitute the entire meaning of the conception*" (Peirce 1965, 5.9). That is, evaluation enters into the enterprise of medical explanation because accounts of disease are immediately focused on controlling and eliminating circumstances judged to be a disvalue. The judgments are in no sense pragmatically neutral. Choosing to call a set of phenomena a disease involves a commitment to medical intervention, the assignment of the sick role, and the enlistment in action of health professionals. To call alcoholism, homosexuality, presbyopia, or minor hookworm infestation diseases, involves judgments closely bound to value judgments. Granted, there is a spectrum from broken limbs to color blindness along which interest in construing a constellation of phenomena as a disease varies. The pain and discomfort of either a broken limb or a schizophrenic break invite immediate medical aid, while issues of color blindness or dissocial behavior lie at the other end of the spectrum. But all along the spectrum, the concept of disease is as much a mode of evaluating as explaining reality.

Commitment to the concept of disease presupposes that there are phenomena physical and mental which can be correlated with events of pain and suffering, so that their patterns can be explained, their courses predicted, and their outcomes influenced favorably. Further, the pain and suffering cannot be the immediate outcome of circumstances which are directly the subject of free choice. They must result from psychological or physiological laws; that is, they must be open to statement in the form of laws, not moral rules. Medicine is the application of scientific, not moral generalizations. Thus, involutional melancholia, duodenal ulcer, and pneumothorax due to gunshot count as diseases, while ignorance, greed, and political violence do not, insofar as the ignorant are capable of learning, the greedy of virtue, and the violent of pacific action. Thus, mental deficiency, kleptomania, and paranoid reactions do count as diseases.

Of course, a broad concept of diseases including both mental and physical models opens one to greater influence by social values. Yet, social judgments are involved in not considering such events as childbirth to be diseases, even though they are associated with considerable morbidity and in fact mortality. Socially desirable goals help draw the lines (King 1954). The same is true with regard to aging and what then counts as disease and health. The acceptable physical state of an 80-year-old would be disease for a 20-year-old Yet, will that always be the case as more can be effected through geriatrics? Diseases are, as Lester King has indicated, patterns which we structure according to our expectations (King 1954).

This is not to argue that confusion between medical and moral issues is not possible or that such confusion is unlikely. Quite the contrary, such confusion is very likely, given the nature of disease. The concept of disease has fuzzy borders with moral concepts. In the 19th century, for example, masturbation was considered to be primarily a physical disease in the same sense that someone now may hold that coronary artery disease is a physical disease though certain forms of stress may be necessary conditions for the disease (Engelhardt 1974b). More alarming examples exist, such as diseases developed to modify political behavior, such as drapetomania, the running away of slaves (Cartwright 1851). Szasz interprets such concepts as a reductio of the use of disease models in psychiatry, rather than as a caveat with regard to confusing compulsive and free action (Szasz 1971). One of Cartwright's contemporary critics was more to the point in his remark that "if a strong desire to do what is wrong be a disease, the violation of anyone of the Ten Commandments will furnish us with a new [disease]…" (Smith 1851, 233). In short, Cartwright's explanation failed because treating runaway slaves as free agents was a better account than treating them as subjects of fugue states.

Of course, one can still use medical force for political ends. Hookworms can be treated to eliminate anemia and thus make citizens more alert, or conceivably, citizens could be drugged into lethargy. The difference is that the first, unlike the second, is focused as well on the autonomy of the individual, his health. The accent of medicine upon liberating individuals from the hindrances of otherwise uncontrollable psychological and physiological forces, is the focus of the concept of health. The concept of health helps define the concept of disease by providing the telos for the medical enterprise. Disease concepts are, as has been argued, pragmatic concepts whose truth is found in action directed to the elimination of illness and toward the establishment of health.

3.3 Health and Disease

Models and accounts of disease are necessarily varied – they focus on the varied, particular limitations to human life. Health, though, represents a direction common to all the continua from particular diseases to wellbeing. If health is a state of freedom from the compulsion of psychological and physiological forces, there is a common leitmotif in the treatment of either schizophrenia or congestive heart failure – namely, the focus on securing the autonomy of the individual from a particular class of restrictions.[1] The unity of models of diseases is found more in the concept of health than in the concept of disease. Health is the common way away from the many ways of disease.

Thus, while the concept of disease is both an evaluatory and explanatory concept, health as a positive concept is more a regulative ideal. This may account in part for the difficulties surrounding attempts to define health operationally, though operational definitions of freedom from particular diseases are more available. Finally, to stress the non-moral character of the concept of health, a reminder from Freud is appropriate: treatment "does not set out to make pathological reactions impossible, but to give the patient… freedom to decide one way or the other" (Freud 1961, 50, n.1.). Medicine, whether in the case of medical or psychological models of disease, is not an enterprise of applied ethics (Engelhardt 1973b), though values influence what limitations on human actions will be considered significant, and at times lead to confusing vices with the compulsions of nature.

In conclusion, health and disease are not symmetrical concepts, nor are they things, though important confusions have arisen from conceiving of them as such. Rather, the concept of disease is a mode of analyzing certain phenomena for the purposes of diagnosis, prognosis, and therapy. The concept is in one respect pragmatic, and in many respects influenced by issues of value. Particular diseases border on questions of moral and political significance. And, while there are many diseases, there is in a sense only one health – a regulative ideal of autonomy directing the physician to the patient as person, the sufferer of the illness, and the reason for all the concern and activity.

References

Albee, George W. 1969. Emerging Concepts of Mental Illness and Models of Treatment: The Psychological Point of View. *American Journal of Psychiatry* 125:870–876.

Broussais, F. J. V. 1821. *Examen des Doctrines Medicales et des Systemes de Nosologie*. Vol. 2. Paris: Mequignon-Marvis.

Cohen, Henry. 1960. In *Concepts of Medicine*, ed. Brandon Lush. Oxford: Pergamon Press.

Constitution of the World Health Organization (Preamble). 1958. *The First Ten Years of the World Health Organization*. Geneva: WHO.

Cartwright, Samuel A. 1851. Report on the Diseases and Physical Peculiarities of the Negro Race. *The New Orleans Medical and Surgical Journal* 7:707–709.

Engelhardt, H. Tristram, Jr. 1973a. *Mind-Body: A Categorial Relation*. The Hague: Martinus Nijhoff.

Engelhardt, H. Tristram, Jr. 1973b. Psychotherapy as Meta-Ethics. *Psychiatry* 36:440–445.

[1] Much is packed in and hidden away in the notion of a "particular class of restrictions" which has only been sketched in part above.

Engelhardt, H. Tristram, Jr. 1974a. Explanatory Models in Medicine: Facts, Theories, and Values. *Texas Reports on Biology and Medicine* 32:225–239.
Engelhardt, H. Tristram, Jr. 1974b. The Disease of Masturbation: Values and the Concept of Disease. *Bulletin of the History of Medicine* 48:234–248.
Faber, Knud. 1923. *Nosography in Modern Internal Medicine*. New York: Paul B. Hoeber.
Feinstein, Alvan R. 1967. *Clinical Judgment*. Baltimore: The Williams and Wilkins Company.
Freud, Sigmund. 1961. *The Standard Edition of the Complete Psychological Works of Sigmund Freud*, ed. and trans. by James Strachey. London: Hogarth Press and The Institute of Psycho-Analysis, Vol. 19, *The Ego and the Id and Other Works*.
Holmes, Thomas H., and Richard H. Rahe. 1967. The Social Readjustment Rating Scale. *Journal of Psychosomatic Research* 11:213–218.
Hudson, Robert P. 1966. The Concept of Disease. *Annals of Internal Medicine* 65.
King, Lester A. 1954. What Is Disease? *Philosophy of Science* 21.
Macklin, Ruth. 1972. Mental Health and Menta! Illness: Some Problems of Definition and Concept Formation. *Philosophy of Science* 39:341–365.
Macklin, Ruth. 1973. The Medical Model in Psychoanalysis and Psychotherapy. *Comprehensive Psychiatry* 14:49–69.
Niebyl, Peter H. 1971. Sennert, van Helmont, and Medical Ontology. *Bulletin of the History of Medicine* 45.
Pagel, Walter. 1958. *Paracelsus*. Basel, Switzerland: S. Karger.
Pagel, Walter. 1944. *The Religious and Philosophical Aspects of van Helmont's Science and Medicine*. Baltimore: The Johns Hopkins Press.
Pagel, Walter, and Marianne Winder. 1968. Harvey and the 'Modern' Concept of Disease. *Bulletin of the History of Medicine* 42:496–509.
Peirce, C. S. 1965. In *Collected Papers*, ed. Charles Hartshorne and Paul Weis, 5.9. Cambridge, Mass: Belknap Press.
Pinel, Philippe. 1798. *Nosographie philosophique, ou la méthode de l'analyse appliqué à la médecine*. Paris: Brosseau.
Romberg, Ernst. 1909. *Lehrbuch der Krankheiten des Herzens und der Blutgefässe*. 2nd ed. Stuttgart: Verlag von Ferdinand Enke.
de Sauvages, Francois Boissier de la Croix. 1768. *Nosologia Methodica, Sistens Morborum Classica. Juxta Sydenhami men ten et Botanicorum Ordinem*. Amsterdam: Fratrum de Tournes.
Siegler, Miriam, and Humphry Osmond. 1973. The 'Sick Role' Revisited. *The Hastings Center Studies* 1:41–58.
Sigerist, Henry E. 1932. *Man and Medicine*., trans. by Margaret G. Boise. New York: W. W. Norton & Co.
Smith, James T. 1851. Review of Dr. Cartwright's Report on the Diseases and Physical Peculiarities of the Negro Race. *The New Orleans Medical and Surgical Journal* 8.
Szasz, Thomas S. 1960. The Myth of Mental Illness. *The American Psychologist* 15:113–118.
Szasz, Thomas S. 1965. *The Ethics of Psychoanalysis*. New York/London: Basic Books, Inc. Publishers.
Szasz, Thomas S. 1971. The Sane Slave. *American Journal of Psychotherapy* 25:228–239.
Temkin, Owsei. 1961. The Scientific Approach to Disease: Specific Entity and Individual Sickness. In *Scientific Change*, ed. A. C. Crombie, 629–647. London: Heinemann.
U. S. National Heart Institute. 1968. *The Framingham Study: An Epidemiological Investigation of Cardiovascular Disease*. Section 1, p. 1b–6. Washington, D.C.: U. S. Government Printing Office.
Virchow, Rudolf. 1895. *Hundert Jahre allgemeiner Pathologie*. Berlin: Verlag von August Hirschwald. English trans. by Lelland J. Rather, *Disease, Life, and Man: Selected Essays by Rudolf Virchow*. 1958. Stanford: Stanford University Press.
Wolf, Stuart. 1961. Disease As a Way of Life: Neural Integration in Systematic Pathology. *Perspectives in Biology and Medicine* 4:288–305.
Wunderlich, Carl A. 1842. Einleitung. *Archiv für physiologische Heilkunde* 1.

Chapter 4
Tracing Philosophy and Medicine Roots: A Focus on Philosophy of Disease

Mary Ann Gardell Cutter

4.1 A Reason to Celebrate

When I was asked to contribute an essay in honor of the 150th volume in the Philosophy and Medicine series, I asked myself, what could a philosopher and clinical ethicist who has spent most of her time teaching undergraduate biomedical ethics say that could contribute to discussions? Ah, herein is the start of an essay. In this essay, and in honor of the Philosophy and Medicine series' 150th volume and 50th anniversary in publishing, I share what I say to my students in the classroom: there is a need for continued dialogue on the mutual dependence of biomedical ethics and philosophy of medicine within a global context. In what follows, I illustrate this mutual dependence of philosophy of medicine and biomedical ethics that is heralded in volumes in the Philosophy and Medicine series. I then illustrate this mutual dependence in discussions of philosophy of disease, a focus of my work for over three-plus decades now. As we celebrate the contributions of the Philosophy and Medicine series, we are reminded of its deep roots and lasting legacy in the literature.

4.2 Situating the Philosophy and Medicine Book Series

As its website says, the Philosophy and Medicine book series is dedicated to the publication of essays and monographs that contribute to scholarship in philosophy of medicine and bioethics. Topics include concepts of health and disease (e.g.,

M. A. G. Cutter (✉)
Department of Philosophy, University of Colorado at Colorado Springs, Colorado Springs, CO, USA
e-mail: mcutter@uccs.edu

L. M. Rasmussen, S. Holm (eds.), *50 Years of Philosophy and Medicine*, Philosophy and Medicine 150, https://doi.org/10.1007/978-3-031-95175-6_4

Nordenfelt et al. 1984), the phenomenology of illness (e.g., Meacham 2015), and ethical topics spanning from womb (e.g., Napier 2011) to tomb (e.g., Taboada 2015). It has sought to create an "intellectual and scholarly focal point that frames the fields of philosophy of medicine and bioethics" (Philosophy and Medicine 2024). The fields have attended to the ontological (i.e., metaphysical or nature-based), epistemological (i.e., knowledge-based), and axiological (i.e., value-based) issues occasioned by thought and practice in medicine and the biomedical sciences. With approximately 150 volumes in print since 1975, "no other series offers as substantial and significant resource for philosophical scholarship regarding issues raised by medicine and the biomedical sciences" (Philosophy and Medicine 2024).

I have been fortunate to be acquainted with the Philosophy and Medicine series since the late 1970s. At that time, and as a student of physician-philosopher Tris Engelhardt (1941–2018) at Georgetown University, I devoured discussions in his "Philosophy of Medicine" class. In the early 1980s, and after a year in biology graduate school, I returned to the study of philosophy of medicine as a graduate student under Dr. Engelhardt. I wanted to continue my philosophical work on disease, following in his scholarship on the subject. During this time at the Center for Ethics and Public Policy at the Baylor College of Medicine, I assisted in organizing Philosophy and Medicine conferences and editing resulting conference papers for publication. Many of the authors that are featured in Philosophy and Medicine series, such as Stuart Spicker, Loretta Kopelman, John Moskop, Corinna Delkeskamp-Hayes, Bill Bondeson, and Mary Rawlinson became influential mentors to me. And there I met George Khushf, Becky White, Lisa Rasmussen, and Mary Cherry, peers whose works I very much admire.

The Philosophy and Medicine book series provides valuable resource materials in philosophy of medicine and bioethics. The body of scholarship in the series provides a forum for an internationally active group of scholars who document the increasing importance of philosophical reflection for multiple dimensions of theory and practice in the health care arena. While it is entitled the "Philosophy and Medicine" series, it draws attention to philosophy *of* medicine and philosophy *in* medicine, as well as medicine *in* philosophy (Carson and Burns 1997; Engelhardt Jr 2022; Marcum 2008). It attends to the dialectical interplay among the elements in the discussion and practice and the importance of involving a range of voices.

There are two trends that drive the continued need for the Philosophy and Medicine book series. First, there has been in the last five decades since Dr. Potter (1970, 1971) (Jonsen 1998), an explosion of interest in one of philosophy of medicine's sub-specialties, biomedical ethics. This explosion has directed interest toward numerous applied issues in health care (e.g., genetic therapy) at the cost of the conceptual ones (e.g., what constitutes proper and beneficial boundaries of human intervention and transformation). This is the case in part because of the contemporary appeal for quick, practical answers to difficult questions and because conceptual presuppositions have been assumed away. A refocusing of attention on issues in the philosophy of medicine is necessary in order to redirect interest to the conceptual approaches informing and framing the practical ones. This is the case because it is our reliance on these approaches that guides our clinical and policy applications.

Second, and in part due to insufficient attention on the conceptual issues that frame biomedical ethical discussions, there is a need for theoretical analysis of topics that traverse borders. These include, but are not limited to, the character of medical theory and practice, the extent to which disease and health are definable, and the "proper" boundaries of medical practice and research in the third millennium. Medicine is no longer a local enterprise. It is framed by professional methodologies and research evidence that are handed down in the medical profession and are reviewed and changed in light of new knowledge and practice, often across national borders (Delkeskamp-Hayes and Cutter 1993). And it is not simply the methodologies and evidence that traverse borders. Determinants of health and disease cross boundaries in an increasing global world, as we experienced during the COVID-19 pandemic (Cutter 2024). As a consequence, topics in philosophy of medicine and biomedical ethics need to be framed within the context of a diverse and changing global culture of medicine, as opposed to a parochial one.

Thus, it is important to have a sense of the field of the philosophy of medicine at large as a broader framework, even if the interest is to focus on select elements in order to address particular issues. In order to respond to these two-fold trends (or concerns), while simultaneously celebrating the richness and diversity of the fields of philosophy of medicine and biomedical ethics, volumes in the Philosophy and Medicine Series take stock of medicine and emerging ethical issues in the broadest sense of the term from philosophical perspectives. Some volumes take on an analytic approach (Sadegh-Zadeh 2011) and others a phenomenological one (Meacham 2015). Some focus on eastern concerns (Fan 2002) and others on western ones (Brody et al. 2009). Some provide a particular religious perspective (Eberl 2017) and others a secular one (Peset and Gracia 1992). Some are more historical (McCullough 1998) and others quite contemporary (Sherlock 2024). Taken together, volumes in the Philosophy and Medicine Series represent shared and disparate views of topics in philosophy of medicine that span cultures. In the onset of a global economy and increased demographic shifts in the world, volumes in the Philosophy and Medicine can serve as tools for discussions across borders regarding how we understand, undertake, and transform the medical human condition.

A central conviction that informs volumes in the Philosophy and Medicine Series is that the older paradigm, when humanities and philosophical reflection were regarded as external and somewhat secondary to medical science and practice, can no longer be sustained. Although the volumes attempt to consider medicine from a philosophical perspective, they are often not rigid to disciplinary perspectives. Some of the authors in the Philosophy and Medicine Series do not have degrees in philosophy. Some do not have degrees in medicine, nursing, or other medical or clinical fields. Taken together, authors in the Philosophy and Medicine Series represent a cross-section of scholars from the international community reflecting on salient topics in philosophy of medicine and the ways in which geographical and cultural boundaries do and do not cross over.

Put another way, while the trends in contemporary medicine are to prioritize biomedical ethics over philosophy of medicine and to offer local perspectives, the Philosophy and Medicine Series has championed conceptual philosophical analysis of the claims and assumptions that frame medicine and clinical practice on a global scale. Authors in the series lay out the terrain of select issues and, when appropriate, develop the connections among the metaphysical, epistemological, and axiological dimensions of the issues set within social contexts. That is, they probe "what is…?," "how do we know…?," and "how do we value….?" in medicine, then or now, and here or there. The intent is sometimes not to provide solutions, but rather to frame the questions and concerns that captivate the attention of medical scientists and practitioners, along with scholars who attend to medical matters. When solutions are offered, they are contextualized within a set of alternative options with the criteria that one could use to make choices, both private and public, and local or global.

Volumes in the Philosophy and Medicine Series are not just publications. They represent a tribe of scholars interested in topics at the intersection of philosophy and medicine. For those of us who have worked on select topics (in my case, philosophy of disease), the Philosophy and Medicine Series has continued to be a source of scholarly research on the nature, knowledge, and value of topics in medicine. My work on disease began with a Philosophy and Medicine publication and has developed through the years. It has focused on how epistemological commitments frame and are framed by ethical ones in the ways in which we classify, describe, explain, diagnose, and treat disease. Let's consider this focus as we illustrate the mutual-dependence of philosophy and medicine and biomedical ethics fostered by work in the Philosophy and Medicine series.

4.3 Philosophy of Disease

While essays on philosophy of disease can be found in journals such as *The Journal of Medicine and Philosophy*, there is a time and place for extended analysis of disease. A study of disease is important because disease is a centralizing notion in health care, one that has direct and important consequences for daily life. How medicine classifies, describes, explains, and diagnoses disease guides treatment (Engelhardt Jr 1996, Chap. 5; Cutter 2003, Chap. 5). It guides what actions are advised to be taken and which ones are not, as well as who is charged with what tasks over what recommended period of time. If one is diagnosed with breast cancer, for instance, there will be certain avenues of treatment (e.g., mastectomy, chemotherapy, radiation) that will be recommended (Cutter 2018, Chap. 4). If one is diagnosed with coronavirus-19, one will not receive treatment recommended for breast cancer but instead a different intervention (Cutter 2024, Chap. 4).

The ways in which we speak of, react to, and experience disease is shaped and directed by a number of interests. These interests, stated philosophically, include metaphysical, epistemological and evaluative ones. They constitute the "language" of disease in that they provide the "grammar" and "rules," so to speak, for constructing meaning about and practical guidelines for addressing what patients bring into the clinic and how it can and *should* be treated. In this way, biomedical ethics needs philosophy of medicine when reflecting upon concepts of disease (also see Khushf 1997).

More specifically, disease is seen through a set of *metaphysical* assumptions, ones that address the question "What is…?." In medicine, defining and explaining what comes into the clinic takes place by providing "facts." The term "fact" is derived from the Latin "factum" (The Complete Oxford English Dictionary 1994, 560) and refers to "a thing done" or a "reality of existence," that is, to something that has really occurred or is actually the case. Such a view assumes that there is a reality "out there" to be discovered, a position called a *realist* view in philosophy. In medicine, a typical test for a fact is verifiability, which seeks to confirm whether the facts correspond to experience. Such a view assumes that matter is the basis of reality, a position called a *materialist* view in philosophy. In clinical medicine, and over time, a materialist view of disease has described a clinical condition in terms of organ systems (e.g., reproductive), individual organs (e.g., breast), tissues (e.g., breast tissue), cells (e.g., breast cells), and molecular components (e.g., biomarkers and genes) (Cutter, 2018, Chap. 3). The position in which objects are reduced to their component parts is known in philosophy as *reductionism*. Here the properties of the whole are the addition or summation of the properties of the individual parts. In the case of breast cancer, the National Cancer Institute describes breast cancer as the abnormal growth and build-up of extra cells in the breast lobes, ducts, tissues, lymph vessels, and lymph nodes that form a mass called a lump or tumor (National Cancer Institute 2024). A tumor is then submitted to pathological tests to determine its size, shape, and, if available, biomarkers and/or genetic characteristics.

The so-called "facts" in medicine are not neutral. They are seen through theoretical frameworks (also see Fleck 1979 [1935]; Cutter 2003, Chaps. 4–6). Descriptions require standardization of terms and, as such, are framed by prior discussions, presumptions, and claims within particular frameworks. For instance, surgeons describe disease in terms of surgical features, geneticists describe them in terms of genetic factors, and pathologists describe them in terms of pathological criteria. Further, such descriptions can and do change. One might think of the change that the American Joint Committee on Cancer (AJCC) Breast Cancer Task Force made from the fifth to the sixth edition in 2003 in recommending that the N (node) category of the TMN (tumor, metastases, node) cancer staging system be changed from one to three categories based on the number of axillary (i.e., under the arm) lymph nodes that are present (American Joint 2010, 423). This change came about in part because of a theoretical shift in understanding the role of lymph nodes in determining the extensiveness of breast cancer and the need for more specific diagnoses of breast cancer so that treatments for breast cancer can be more precise.

Given that the so-called "facts" of medicine are not neutral, it may be misleading to say that disease is "out there" to be discovered as reducible matter. Rather, disease in part reflects the "lenses" through which a clinical knower views and manipulates this so-called reality. Disease is in part the experience of a disability, dysfunction, and/or suffering reported by a patient that hinders the achievement of certain goals. On this *idealist* view of reality, disease may not be fully reducible to matter that can be studied using laboratory tests. It is not a thing but an idea of a *holistic* event in the life of a patient. For instance, breast cancer reflects not simply a collection of mutated cells that affects biological function in certain ways; it constitutes an experience reported by a patient in the context of his, her, and their life (Cutter 2018, Chap. 5).

Further, the "facts" of disease are structured in terms of *epistemological* claims and assumptions. In this way, disease is an explanatory concept and, as such, brings coherence to the multiplicity of events we encounter in medicine (Cutter, 2003, Chap. 4). It brings coherence to the signs and symptoms that bring patients into the clinic, and the pathoanatomical and pathophysiological data that are generated by laboratory findings by gathering and interpreting empirical data within the framework of interpretations that have been handed down and serve as clinical standards. In that disease brings coherence to the signs and symptoms that patients bring into the clinic, it is a *rationalist* concept. It accounts for orderly patterns of events according to the laws of science and medicine. In that disease brings coherence to a set of medical data, it is an *empiricist* concept. It brings sense and meaning to the empirical data that is gathered by clinical investigators. Here clinical facts are verified by repeatable experiments and data and they maintain an accepted status until they are shown to be non-verifiable. And should this occur, the interpretation of clinical facts changes.

In this epistemic approach, disease relates "two worlds of observations" (Engelhardt Jr 1996, 209), the world of the clinic and the world of the laboratory. The findings of the clinician are related to the observations of the pathoanatomists and pathophysiologists and take on a new significance through these anatomical and pathological observations. For instance, molecular science shows us that breast cancer is no longer a single disease. Breast cancer is now understood in terms of Estrogen-Positive, HER2-Positive, Triple-Negative, and BRCA frames of reference, among others (Cutter 2018, Chap. 2). With these shifts, what results is an expansion of the epistemic or explanatory powers of medicine and the ability to diagnose and treat clinical problems with greater accuracy or precision. Therein lies the hope of precision or personalized medicine today.

Third, disease is an *evaluative* concept (Cutter 2003, Chaps. 6 and 7). To see a phenomenon as a disease, illness, or disability is to see something wrong with it. Disease is experienced as a failure to achieve an expected state, a state held to be proper to the person afflicted. This may be a failure to achieve an expected freedom from pain or suffering, an expected level of function or ability, a realization of human form or grace, and/or an expected span of life. This may also be a failure to achieve a state requested by a patient, determined to be beneficial to a patient, and/or in keeping with the standards of ethical integrity and the moral virtues of the health care profession. In other words, the "facts" of disease are inextricably tied to the "value" of disease and its treatment, where value is understood as an important and enduring sign of significance or worth, belief, or ideal that guides action or intention.

The topic of the extent to which disease is a value-neutral vs. a value-ladened concept has received much attention in the Philosophy and Medicine literature (e.g., Engelhardt and Spicker 1975; Wulff 1981; Nordenfelt et al. 1984; Reznek 1987;

Stempsey 2000; Cutter 2003, Chaps. 6 and 7). Disease is an evaluative concept because disease is not simply a "fact." It entails judgments concerning what actions *ought* to be taken, including trade-offs between beneficial and harmful outcomes and respect for ethical boundaries that cannot be compromised. Consider the case of ductal carcinoma in situ (Cutter 2018, Chap. 4). Ductal carcinoma in situ is marked by notable cellular mutations that, if left untreated, may grown further and metastasize or leave the breast area. Ductal carcinoma in situ is typically not painful and may not metastasize beyond the breast ducts. But it may, and if it does, it could lead to significant harm to the patient, including death. As a consequence, cases of ductal carcinoma in situ, as well as early states of hyperplasia in breast cells, may be the focus of clinical interventions because, all things considered, they are disvalued and might be harmful to a patient.

A related issue is the clinical determination of what is considered "normal" and "abnormal." "Normal" and "abnormal" are recognized as such within a particular context of explanations and evaluation. Because the measure of an individual organ, tissue, or cell is highly uninformative, a clinician has no idea from a single case what range of data can count as "normal" or "abnormal." Group data must be taken into account. What is needed is a range of measurements for a range of populations that clinicians and researchers can agree upon that constitutes "normal" or "abnormal." Here, "normal" can mean that which is statistical, average or mean, typical or expectable, conducive to the survival of a species, innocuous or harmless, commonly aspired to, or excellent in its class (Murphy 1976, 117–133). In some sense, hyperplasia in breast cells is "normal" in that it is a common preneoplastic response to stimulus, leading to benign (noncancerous) cellular growth. Alternatively, "abnormal" can mean what is statistical, average, not typical, not conducive to the survival of a species, harmful, not commonly aspired to, or deficient in its class. In some cases, hyperplasia in breast cells can lead to malignant or cancerous tumors. The determination of what is "normal" and "abnormal" requires value judgments about thresholds between and among points of data. In medicine, such judgments typically concern the ethical values of how to maximize patient welfare and minimize patient harm, respect patient choices, and allocate limited medical resources.

Taken together, the metaphysical, epistemological, and evaluative dimensions of disease operate within *social contexts* (Cutter 2003, Chap. 8). The diagnosis of a disease takes place within the social practices of developing professional clinical standards, devising educational requirements and licensure agreements, formulating funding options, and instituting health laws and policies. To claim that a patient has a disease is to cast that individual in social roles where certain societal responses are expected (Parsons 1958). Some of the social responses include assigning individuals a sick role, expecting that such persons seek help from socially recognized professionals, excusing sick persons from responsibilities for certain tasks while recovering from disease conditions, and expecting that care for certain diseases is covered by medical insurance plans and is protected by particular health care policies. For instance, choices to divide stages and sub-divide breast cancer stages and grades into a certain number turn on cost-benefit calculations and understandings of prudent actions that have direct implications for the ways patients are treated within the social contexts of insurance practices, employee benefits, and the protection of vulnerable individuals in a society.

Put another way, the social context of our understanding and treatment of disease matters. It matters not tangentially, but at its core. In the United States, for instance, a study shows that "[b]lack women with breast cancer … are on average about 40% more likely to die of the disease than white women with breast cancer" (Parker-Pope 2024; also see Torres et al. 2024). Another study shows that those who are economically challenged tend not to request or know about reconstruction options after a mastectomy (Doheny 2014). Another study shows that there is a lack of standards for survivorship care in breast cancer medicine, including a lack of treatment of postsurgical pain and immobility, infertility care, and general follow-up care for women with breast cancer (Salz 2013). Understanding how social forces frame clinical classifications, descriptions, and choices is critical in order to uncover assumptions and claims in breast cancer medicine. Such a move opens up doors to research questions and understandings that may address problems in treating breast cancer that we currently face.

The metaphysical, epistemological, and evaluative dimensions of disease within social contexts are not separate and distinct, but rather frame and limit each other (Cutter 2018, Chap. 6). Facts are method-ladened, the fact/method dyads are evaluative, and the fact/method/value triads are socially framed. In classifying breast cancer, for instance, a decision has to be made regarding how many cells with deviant changes of a certain kind in the biopsied breast tissue must be present before the cells are labeled as "carcinoma" or "cancer." An explanation is given about the relation between the mutating cells and breast cancer classifications and descriptions. To be too liberal in classifying cells as "cancer" will lead to unnecessary treatment, which harms patients, undermines patient autonomy, and wastes resources. To be too conservative in the classification will lead to delayed treatment, which leads to increased pain and suffering, as well as unnecessary deaths among women. On this view, the lines among "benign," "suspicious," and "cancer," as well as Stage 0 through 4 in breast cancer classification, are in part discovered and in part created. The lines among who gets clinical care and who does not, and who lives and who dies, are in part discovered and in part created. They involve explicit and implicit appeals to fact/method/value triads within social frames of reference.

4.4 Some Thoughts on Where to Go

This essay has focused on a need for continued dialogue on the mutual dependence of biomedical ethics and philosophy of medicine within a global context. Through some case studies, it has illustrated a mutual dependence of philosophy of medicine and biomedical ethics that is heralded in volumes in the Philosophy and Medicine series. As we celebrate the contributions of the Philosophy and Medicine series, we are reminded of its lasting legacy in the literature, and the need for such. On this point, where might one go from here?

For me, a legacy of the Philosophy and Medicine series points me in the direction of focusing more on intersectionality in medicine. *Intersectionality* is originally a sociological framework that makes sense of the impact of power structures and macro-level discrimination on individual identities and social identities, including gender, sex, race, ethnicity, caste, class (economic status), religion (spirituality), disability, height, weight, physical appearance, and age (Cutter 2012). These intersections and overlapping social identities may be both empowering and oppressing. They can be empowering when such identities are dominant in a culture, such as when someone shares the identities of the dominant culture or trend. The intersections and overlapping social identities can be oppressing when one's identities are disenfranchised or a target of prejudice (i.e., biased thinking) and discrimination (i.e., biased actions against a group of people).

Intersectionality arises out of the work of feminists at the end of the twentieth century. Civil rights advocate and legal scholar Kimberlé Williams Crenshaw (1989) introduces the idea of "intersectionality" to demonstrate how such dimensions frame the lives of black women and the discrimination and oppression that they experience in terms of their interlocking racial and gendered identities. Her work is ground-breaking as she shows that a focus on a single dimension of identity (e.g., gender) fails to explain the context in which individuals make choices in a culture. Multiple dimensions (e.g., gender, race, and class) are needed. Writer Audre Lorde, a self-proclaimed black, lesbian, mother, warrior, poet, and breast cancer patient, detailed her life in "a country where racism, sexism, and homophobia are inseparable" (Lorde 2007 [1984], 110) and the prejudice and discrimination that she experienced as someone who lives among the borders of multiple identities, some of which are disempowering. And, yes, this was the case for her as a breast cancer patient in the clinical setting before her death in 1992.

According to feminist sociologist Kathy Davis, intersectionality has two distinct characteristics. First, intersectionality unpacks "effects of race, class, and gender on women's identities, experience, and struggles for empowerment" (Davis 2008, 71). It shows how identities of difference impact and are impacted by experiences of power, prejudice, and discrimination. Such is the focus of Crenshaw's work. Second, according to Davis, intersectionality assists in deconstructing the "binary opposition and universalism inherent in the modernist paradigms of Western philosophy and science" (Davis 2008, 71). An intersectional account reveals how assumptions and claims about how we know, what we know, and what and how we value generate, shape, and maintain explicit and implicit binary oppositions and universal paradigms in thinking and practice. Classifying each other in terms of the binaries of male/female, black/white, rich/poor, and old/young contributes to systems of power and oppression that need to be dismantled if we are to interact with one another in a way that breaks down the "haves" from the "have-nots."

For instance, during the COVID-19 pandemic (Cutter 2024), individuals from particular populations (e.g., the elderly; members of particular racial, ethnic, and economic groups; the uninsured) were more likely to contract COVID-19, become sick from it, and die from it. As Meredith Freed and her colleagues at the Kaiser Family Foundation report, "[a]s of the week ending October 1, 2022, the United

States has lost nearly 1.1 million lives to COVID-19, of which about 790,000 are people ages 65 and older. People 65 and older account for 16% of the total US population but 75% of all COVID deaths to date" (Freed et al. 2022). Further, Black, Hispanic, AIAN (Alaskan Native), and NHOPI (Native Hawaiian and Other Pacific Islander) people were more likely to contract COVID-19 and suffer debilitating consequences. As Latoya Hill and Samantha Artiga report, "[a]s of August 5, 2022, the Centers for Disease Control and Prevention (CDC) reported a total of over 84 million cases, for which race/ethnicity was known for 65% or over 55 million, and a total of over 880,000 deaths, for which race/ethnicity was known for 85% or over 750,000" (Hill and Artiga 2022). Still further, individuals who lacked insurance were more vulnerable to COVID-19. As Stan Dorn and Rebecca Gordan report, "[n]ationally, roughly 1 out of every 3 COVID-19 deaths are linked to health insurance gaps. More than 40% of all COVID-19 infections are associated with health insurance gaps. By August 31, 2020, health insurance gaps were linked to an estimated 2.6 million COVID-19 cases and 58,000 COVID-19 deaths. By February 1, 2021, 10.9 million infections and 143,000 COVID-19 deaths may have been associated with health insurance gaps" (Dorn and Gordon 2021). During the COVID-19 pandemic, factors, including lower mean income, lack of proper housing, frontline jobs in the low-income essential category that precluded working from home, lack of private transportation, and the absence of employment-linked healthcare benefits, contributed to a stark divide between who lived and who died, and who got sick and who were protected. Identities of difference mattered during the pandemic, and our responses were less than attentive to systems of power that influenced individual and public health outcomes. We can only hope that more work focuses on what we can learn from our actions and inactions during the COVID-19 pandemic.

One can think about intersectional thinking and action in terms of the intersection of dimensions of identity and practice that create and sustain systems of power and oppression in a culture. Here, cultural dimensions, systematic factors, relationality, personal contextual factors, and the "isms" in our cultures (e.g., racism, sexism, homophobia, ageism, classism, ableism, religious and spiritual intolerance) intersect to create contexts in need of recognition and study. In medicine, for instance, such influences make a difference between who is heard in the clinic and who is not, who is diagnosed and who is not, who is treated and who is not, and who lives and who dies, and in what ways. Such contexts raise conceptual and ethical issues that may not be acknowledged and acted upon if not for reflections on the assumptions and claims that frame medical thought and action. Herein lies the important contributions of volumes in the Philosophy and Medicine series.

In this way, more work is needed on an intersectional account of disease. It can assist in making explicit assumptions and claims that frame an understanding of a particular disease. It can call into question such assumptions and claims. It can look more closely at which populations of patients are more vulnerable to the harms, including death, from particular disease conditions. This can serve as guidance in clinical practice as well as research. While the COVID-19 pandemic is (sort of) behind us and breast cancer medicine has significantly evolved, there will be another pandemic and certain populations of women are more vulnerable to breast cancer than others. It's time do to better, and discussions about such matters drawn from those who engage in dialogue at the threshold of medicine and philosophy can assist in guiding such questions and responses.

On this note, I conclude with celebrating the contributions of those who have written in the Philosophy and Medicine book series and those who carry the series into the third millennium. There is much to do, and with the work of those committed to such dialogues, I am confident that discussions will continue and we will be able to continue to celebrate the lasting legacy of the Philosophy and Medicine book series.

References

American Joint Committee on Cancer. 2010. *AJCC Cancer Staging Handbook*. Springer.

Brody, Howard A., Zahra Meghan, and Kimberly Greenwald, eds. 2009. *Michael Ryan's Writing on Medical Ethics*. Springer Nature.

Carson, Ronald A., and Chester R. Burns. 1997. *Philosophy of Medicine and Bioethics*. Kluwer.

Crenshaw, Kimberlé Williams. 1989. Demarginalizing the Intersection of Race and Sex: A Black Feminist Critique of Antidiscrimination Doctrine, Feminist Theory, and Antiracist Politics. *University of Chicago Legal Forum* 14:538–554.

Cutter, Mary Ann G. 2003. *Reframing Disease Contextually*. Kluwer Academic Publishers.

Cutter, Mary Ann G. 2012. *The Ethics of Gender-Specific Disease*. Routledge.

Cutter, Mary Ann G. *Thinking Through Breast Cancer: A Philosophical Exploration of Diagnosis, Treatment, and Survival*. Oxford University Press, 2018.

Cutter, Mary Ann G. 2024. *An Ethics of Clinical Uncertainty: Lessons from the COVID-19 Pandemic*. Routledge.

Davis, Kathy. 2008. Intersectionality as Buzzword: A Sociology of Science Perspective on What Makes a Feminist Theory Successful. *Feminist Theory* 9:67–85.

Delkeskamp-Hayes, Corinna, and Mary Ann Gardell Cutter, eds. 1993. *Science, Technology, and the Art of Medicine*. Kluwer Academic Publishers.

Doheny, Kathleen. 2014. Many Women Who Have Mastectomy Don't Get Breast Reconstruction. *Health. U.S. News. Com.*

Dorn, Stan, and Rebecca Gordon. 2021. The Catastrophic Cost of Uninsurance: COVID-19 Cases and Deaths Closely Tied to America's Health Coverage Gaps. *Families USA: The Voice for Health Care Consumers*. March 4. https://familiesusa.org/resources/the-catastrophic-cost-of-uninsurance-covid-19-cases-and-deaths-closely-tied-to-americas-health-coverage-gaps/.

Eberl, Jason T. 2017. *Contemporary Controversies in Catholic Bioethics*. Springer Nature.

Engelhardt, H. Tristram, Jr. 1996. *Foundations of Bioethics*. 2nd ed. Oxford University Press.

Engelhardt, H. Tristram Jr The Philosophy of Medicine: Framing the Field. Kluwer Academic Publishers, 2022.

Engelhardt, H. Tristram, Jr., and Stuart F. Spicker. 1975. *Explanation and Evaluation in the Biomedical Sciences*. Kluwer Academic Publishers.

Fan, Ruiping. 2002. *Confucian Bioethics*. Kluwer Academic Publishers.

Fleck, Ludwik. *Genesis and Development of a Scientific Fact,* edited by T.J. Trenn and R.K. Merton and translated by F. Bradley and T.J. Trenn. University of Chicago Press, 1979. [1935].

Freed, Meredith, Trisha Neuman, Jennifer Kates, and Juliette Cubanski. 2022. Deaths Among Older Adults Due to COVID-19 Jumped During the Summer of 2022 Before Falling Somewhat in September. *KFF*. October 6. https://www.kff.org/coronavirus-covid-19/issue-brief/deaths-among-older-adults-due-to-covid-19-jumped-during-the-summer-of-2022-before-falling-somewhat-in-september.

Hill, Latoya, and Samantha Artiga. 2022. COVID-19 Cases and Deaths by Race/Ethnicity: Current Data and Changes Over Time. *KFF*. August 22. https://www.kff.org/coronavirus-covid-19/issue-brief/covid-19-cases-and-deaths-by-race-ethnicity-current-data-and-changes-over-time.

Jonsen, Albert R. 1998. *The Birth of Bioethics*. Oxford University Press.

Khushf, George. 1997. Why Bioethics Needs the Philosophy of Medicine: Some Implications of Reflection on Concepts of Health and Disease. *Theoretical Medicine and Bioethics* 18:145–163.

Lorde, Audre. 2007. *Sister Outsider: Essays and Speeches*. Crossing Press.

Marcum, James A. 2008. *An Introductory Philosophy of Medicine: Humanizing Modern Medicine*. Springer.

McCullough, Laurence B. 1998. *John Gregory's Writing on Medical Ethics and Philosophy of Medicine*. Kluwer Academic Publishers.

Meacham, Darian, ed. 2015. *Medicine and Society: New Continental Perspectives*. Springer Nature.

Murphy, Edmond. 1976. *The Logic of Medicine*. Johns Hopkins University Press.

Napier, Stephen. 2011. *Persons, Moral Worth, and Embryos*. Springer Nature.

National Cancer Institute. 2024. *National Institutes of Health*. What You Need to Know About Breast Cancer. Maryland: National Cancer Institute. http://www.cancer.gov/publications/patient-education/WYNTK_breast.pdf.

Nordenfelt, Lennart, B. Ingemar, and B. Lindahl, eds. 1984. *Health, Disease, and Causal Explanations in Medicine*. D. Reidel Publishing Company.

Parker-Pope, Tara. 2024. The Breast Cancer Racial Gap. *New York Times*. March 3. https://well.blogs.nytimes.com/2014/03/03/the-breast-cancer-racial-gap.

Parsons, Talcott. 1958. Definitions of Health and Illness in the Light of American Values and Social Structures. In *Patient's Physicians, and Illness*, ed. E. G. Jaco, 167–187. The Free Press.

Peset, José Luis, and Diego Gracia. 1992. *The Ethics of Diagnosis*. Kluwer Academic Publishers.

Philosophy and Medicine. 2024. *Philosophy and Medicine Book Series*. Springer. https://www.springer.com/series/6414?srsltid=AfmBOoo-j6Y9hy5CHTkixS6QSM2Y23JoDLS7_9glK_eTnCkp7xnevWVQ.

Potter, Van Rensselaer. 1970. Bioethics: The Science of Survival. *Perspectives in Biology and Medicine* 14:127–153.

Potter, Van Rensselaer. 1971. *Bioethics: Bridge to the Future*. Prentice-Hall.

Reznek, Lawrie. 1987. *The Nature of Disease*. Routledge and Kegan Paul.

Sadegh-Zadeh, Kazem. 2011. *Handbook of Analytic Philosophy of Medicine*. Springer Nature.

Salz, Talya. 2013. *Survivorship Care Plans in Research and Practice. CA: A Cancer Journal for Clinicians*. http://www.ncbi.nlm.nih.gov/pmc/articles/pmc3330140.

Sherlock, Richard. 2024. *Medicine and Hope: A Natural Theology of Human Caretaking*. Springer Nature.

Stempsey, William E. 2000. *Disease and Diagnosis: Value-dependent Realism. Kluwer*.

Taboada, Paulina. 2015. *Sedation at the End-of-Life: An Interdisciplinary Approach*. Springer Nature.

The Complete Oxford English Dictionary. 1994. Clarendon Press.

Torres, Juliana, et al. 2024. Racial Differences in Breast Cancer Survival Between Black and White Women According to Tumor Subtype: A Systematic Review and Meta-Analysis. *Journal of Clinical Oncology*. 42 (32): 3867–3879. https://doi.org/10.1200/JCO.23.02311.

Wulff, Henrik R. 1981. *Rational Diagnosis and Treatment: An Introduction to Clinical Decision-Making*. 2nd ed. Blackwell Scientific Publications.

Chapter 5
Phenomenology of Health and Illness in the American-English Tradition

Fredrik Svenaeus

5.1 Introduction

Kay Toombs' *The Meaning of Illness: A Phenomenological Account of the Different Perspectives of Physician and Patient* (1992) is not the first book in the series of *Philosophy and Medicine* to contain chapters referring to and making use of works in the phenomenological tradition. You find phenomenological perspectives in chapters published in earlier volumes of the series, mainly addressing questions related to the status and nature of the lived body, that is: the body as the point of view of everyday experience in contrast to the body as a biological organism.[1] However, to my best knowledge, Toombs' book it is the first monograph – not only in this series but in the English language – to deal explicitly with the phenomenology of illness, and, also, to relate this perspective of the patient to the medical encounter and the point of view of the physician.[2] In her endeavor, Toombs makes

[1] Other early books in the series containing phenomenological pieces include: S. F. Spicker (Ed.), *Organism, Medicine and Metaphysics. Essays in Honor of Hans Jonas on his 75th Birthday* (no. 7). (1978); R. M. Zaner (Ed.), *Death: Beyond Whole-Brain Criteria* (no. 31). (1988); and D. Leder (Ed.), *The Body in Medical Thought and Practice* (no. 43). (1992). Toombs' book was published simultaneously with the book by Leder: S. K. Toombs, *The Meaning of Illness: A Phenomenological Account of the Different Perspectives of Physician and Patient* (no. 42). (1992).

[2] Four important early works in the English-Speaking tradition of phenomenology of medicine that deserve to be mentioned here are: R. M. Zaner, *The Context of Self: A Phenomenological Inquiry Using Medicine as a Clue.* (1981); H. Jonas, *The Imperative of Responsibility: In Search of Ethics for the Technological Age.* (1984); D. Leder, *The Absent Body.* Chicago: (1990); and E. J. Cassell, *The Nature of Suffering*. (1991).

F. Svenaeus (✉)
Centre for Studies in Practical Knowledge, Södertörn University, Huddinge, Sweden
e-mail: fredrik.svenaeus@sh.se

L. M. Rasmussen, S. Holm (eds.), *50 Years of Philosophy and Medicine*,
Philosophy and Medicine 150, https://doi.org/10.1007/978-3-031-95175-6_5

use of arguments found in works by first-generation German and French phenomenologists, including works containing attempts to deal with the topic of phenomenology of health and illness, which is, as a matter of fact, a rather rare topic in the phenomenological tradition.[3]

5.2 Toombs' Proposal for a Phenomenology of Illness

The chapter on "Illness" is number two in Toombs' book, preceded by a Chap. 1 on "The separate worlds of physician and patient," and followed by a Chap. 3 on "The body" and a Chap. 4 on "The healing relationship" (Toombs 1992). Toombs' strategy is to show how different in form and content the worlds of physicians and patients are and that this difference depends on the focus on disease versus illness. Physicians study the body of the patient as a biological organism out of order due to functional failures caused by disease processes (or by injuries or congenital defects). They live in a world defined by diagnostic hypotheses, bodily examinations, laboratory tests and treatment possibilities. Patients, in contrast, live in a world of personally experienced illness, a world full of pain, bodily impairments, everyday problems, and anxiety about the future brought about by the changed life situation.

How can these two radically different worlds be brought into contact with one another? According to Toombs, not primarily by way of patients learning more about medical diagnoses and disease processes, but by way of physicians learning and understanding more about what it means to be ill. The way to do this is not only to become more empathic and interested in what the patient feels and thinks. To learn and understand more about the patient's life situation and personal narrative are, indeed, key moves in becoming a better doctor, but what Toombs also wants to show is that the tradition of phenomenology can help doctors understand what the experience of illness consists in and how it is different from, although related to, having a body wrought by diseases.

To achieve this, Toombs turns to four classic phenomenologists: Edmund Husserl, Alfred Schutz, Jean-Paul Sartre, and Maurice Merleau-Ponty. Husserl helps her to put into play the concepts of subjectivity, intentionality, horizon, life world, and temporality, whereas Schutz provides her with resources to tell apart the different worlds of physician and patient in terms of their specific objects and projects. Sartre's phenomenology is made use of to better understand the processes of

[3] Two examples of phenomenologists of illness that Toombs mentions in her book are Herbert Plügge and Jan Hendrik van den Berg (two others that she could have mentioned are Friedrich Buytendijk and Victor-Emil von Gebsattel). If one considers not only somatic medicine, but also the tradition of German and French psychopathology in the 20th century, there are many other phenomenologists of illness to be included on the list: Karl Jaspers, Ludwig Binswanger, Eugène Minkowski, and Erwin Straus, to mention just a few (Straus also published works in English after having emigrated to the USA in 1938 for political reasons).

illness and how they are related to attaining a different point of view on your own body. Merleau-Ponty, finally, is used to fine-tune the phenomenology of the body that we need to fully understand illness and how it is related to disease. The counterpart of illness – health – is not addressed by Toombs – but I will return to health when discussing other phenomenological approaches to medical matters below.

So how is illness experienced according to Toombs? What is "the meaning of illness," to quote the title of her book? In summing up her analysis, she writes:

> The fundamental level is that of pre-reflective sensory experience. At this level one's immediate experience is such that it leads one to become aware of some disruption in the manner in which one "exists" one's body. That is, some unusual sensory experience (such as pain, weakness, or some visual apprehension of an alteration in body) causes the patient to shift attention from ongoing involvements in projects in the world and to focus upon the bodily disruption. Once the immediate experience of disruption is thematized at the reflective level, it may be apprehended as "suffered illness." "Suffered illness" is a synthetic totality in that it incorporates the immediate bodily sensations – the various and varied aches and pains – as part of a larger whole. . . . At a further interpretive level the patient apprehends "suffered illness" to be "disease." The lived body becomes objectified as a neurophysiological organism and the immediate sensory disruption is apprehended as a particular illness (Toombs 1992: 38).

At this point, it should perhaps be mentioned that Toombs suffers from a particular illness herself, an illness with a specific diagnostic name: multiple sclerosis (MS). The phenomenological description of how the patterns of pre-reflective experience are gradually changed in falling ill, forcing the sufferer to focus attention on her own body because of weakness and numbness, which in turn give rise to an experience of the suffered illness itself, and diagnostic hypotheses about disease processes, fits very well with the onset and ongoing experience of MS. When the sufferer turns to health care and meets with a physician, illness can finally be transformed into a medical diagnosis by way of scientific investigations and a name having to do with the bodily processes involved (in the case of MS rather with the end state of the disease process, namely scars – sclerosis – formed as a result of the loss of myelin normally protecting nerve fibers.)

To be diagnosed by a doctor is the final interpretative level of falling ill, according to Toombs. However, to receive a medical diagnosis will certainly not by itself lead to abatement of bodily symptoms, they stay, and sometimes become worse, as do the life world problems and existential reflections brought on by illness. What could lead to the ease of suffering is rather medical treatment alternatives induced by way of the diagnosis. Consequently, the four-stage temporal process of illness suffering put in place by Toombs, with the aid of Sartre, continues to contain elements of all four stages: pre-reflective sensory experience, illness suffering, disease pondering, and disease by way of a diagnosis received from the physician.[4]

---

[4] Other phenomenologists of illness have further fine-tuned Sartre's model, see Svenaeus (2009).

5.3 Phenomenology and the Medical Encounter

In some cases, being told a diagnosis may lead to relief when the scientific explanation becomes entrenched in the experience of the ill person: it hurts and is bothersome, but I know what it is, and it is not dangerous (arthritis). In other cases, the diagnosis will make the suffering worse because I learn that I am suffering from a life-threatening condition (breast cancer). The example of MS is somewhat in between – the disease is chronic and often gets worse with time, but it may progress slowly, and much has to do with if the patient can compensate for the symptoms and reorganize her everyday life patterns. Diabetes is a similar example of a chronic disease, but in this case, there is even more room for personal reflection and change of everyday habits to influence the experience of illness and the progress of the disease.

Doctors may play an important supportive role in this process of getting accustomed to a different form of life with chronic disease and not losing hope. A lot has to do with how the physician addresses the patient in the first encounter and if he tries to learn about her fears and thoughts about the diagnosis in question. Toombs writes:

> A few days earlier I had fortuitously read an article in a popular magazine in the doctor's office which related the story of a young woman (a former beauty queen), stricken with M.S., who was now severely disabled and confined to a wheelchair. Consequently, on hearing the diagnosis, my first question was, "Will I end up in a wheelchair?" The physician replied that unfortunately he could give me no guarantees for the future. Not unnaturally I interpreted this response to mean that I would indeed become disabled and perhaps in the near future (Toombs 1992: 45).

Toombs goes on to point out that if the physician had been attentive to her preunderstanding of the illness in question, he could have "acted as an arbiter of meaning – perhaps enabling the patient to modify or change an inappropriate interpretation of the situation" (Toombs 1992: 45). This would have been very valuable for her and could considerably have eased her suffering. But the physician in question was mainly focused on providing accurate *information* about how the disease might progress, anxious to offer any promises that could later lead to a questioning of his scientific competence. In this way, he was not focused on *her*, but on the disease process and the fear to carry responsibility. It would have been very helpful if he had at least pointed out to her that it may be a long time before she needed to make use such equipment, and, even more helpful, if he had asked her about why she came up with this very question about becoming bound to a wheelchair.

In the two following chapters of the book, Toombs further examines the different aspects of embodiment involved in the illness experiences and the attitudes formed towards the body in the medical encounter. She also mentions the possibilities of empathy and illness narratives to connect the two different worlds of doctor and patient and employs the terminology of a "healing relationship" (Toombs 1992: 110). All of these three strategies will develop into major alternatives for better health care in the 1990s and early 2000s, keywords being "clinical empathy"

(Decety 2012), "narrative medicine" (Charon 2006), and, attached to the healing relationship, the notions of "patient-" and "person-centered care" (Marcum et al. 2017).

5.4 Phenomenology of Medicine in the Contemporary Context

Phenomenology of medicine significantly expands in the English-speaking context during the 1990s and early 2000s, and Toombs herself has edited the volume in the *Philosophy & Medicine* series which is most emblematic of this development: *Handbook of Phenomenology and Medicine*, containing further explorations on the themes that she introduced in her 1992 book by no less than 24 authors (Toombs 2001). In the 2000s and 2010s we have seen a lively discussion in journals and book volumes on phenomenology of medicine themes, not least connected to feminist and disability studies, but also to bioethics in a broader sense (Svenaeus 2017). It is not possible to present an overview of this many-facetted literature in a single chapter, so I will instead focus on the narrower theme of the second chapter of Toombs' book presented above: phenomenology of illness (Toombs 1992: Chap. 2). In many ways this theme is not only the heart and core of Toombs' book but also of phenomenology of medicine as such. In contrast to medical science, the phenomenology of medicine returns to the *experiences* of illness endured by persons, the happenings that make diseases worth exploring in the first place, looking for ways to cease or ease suffering. That medical therapies are not the only thing that can make life better for patients is yet an important reason for turning to phenomenology of illness, much depends on how the patient lives with and interprets her bodily ailments, as Toombs points out in her book.

A large slice of contemporary phenomenology of medicine has been devoted to developing an account of health and illness that proceeds from the first-person perspective when attempting to understand the ill person in contrast to and connection with the third-person perspective on diseases. This first-person perspective includes what we may call a second-person perspective – that is, the perspective of the health-care practitioner meeting with the patient in attempting to understand and heal. Roughly, it is possible to discern two contemporary proposals for how to conceptualize health and illness in the literature following Toombs' 1992 book: the one proceeding mainly from the philosophy of Maurice Merleau-Ponty with Drew Leder (2016, 2024) and Havi Carel (2008, 2016) as main proponents, and the one proceeding from Martin Heidegger with Kevin Aho (2008, 2018), and Fredrik Svenaeus (2017, 2022) as main advocates.

The essential idea of the first proposal is that illness consists in an appearance of the own-body as conspicuous, obtrusive, or obstinate in the activities of the afflicted person, much in line with Toombs' observations. This is not a question regarding maladies present in the physical body of the person – the body as it appears from the third-person perspective of medical science. Every human experience is embodied and from the phenomenological perspective this means that the body is a person's point of view and way of experiencing and understanding every part and thing of the world (Merleau-Ponty 2012). Not only can I experience my own body as an object of my experience – when I feel it or touch it or look at it in the mirror – but the body is also that which makes a person's experiences possible in the first place. The *lived body* (in contrast to the physical body) is an intentional arc – a body schema – that makes it possible for me to exist in space and time and experience a world shared with other persons (Gallagher 2005; Slatman 2014).

The second proposal acknowledges this pivotal role of the lived body in falling ill, but emphasizes that illness amounts to finding oneself in an alienating *mood* that involves the whole *world* of the suffering person (Heidegger 1996; Ratcliffe 2008). The difference between the two proposals is mainly one of emphasis and terminology, since the version found in Leder and Carel certainly also involves the life-world matters and existential themes present in Aho and Svenaeus. We should also mention here the English translation of a collection of essays by Hans-Georg Gadamer with the title *The Enigma of Health* (1996). Gadamer's approach to health in this volume immediately attracted quite a few readers in the fields of philosophy of medicine and medical ethics – because of his fame and standing in the continental tradition of philosophy – and have been important for Aho and Svenaeus in developing more substantial health theories on Heideggerian ground. The essays by Gadamer were originally published or presented as talks in the 1970s and 1980s, but in the German speaking context of phenomenology of medicine and psychiatry, which, as mentioned above, has attracted very little attention in the English-speaking world.

As Toombs' analysis makes clear, the phenomenon of illness is far more concrete and easier to get hold of than the phenomenon of health. When we are ill, life is often penetrated by feelings of confusion, helplessness, pain, nausea, fear, dizziness, fatigue, or difficulties to breath or move one's body. Health, in contrast, effaces itself in an enigmatic way. It seems to be the absence of every such feeling of illness, the state or process which we are in when everything is flowing smoothly, running the usual way without hindrance. But is illness our only possibility for phenomenological analysis? Cannot health itself be explicated phenomenologically?[5] Gadamer, in the book mentioned above, *The Enigma of Health*, takes this to be the case:

> So what possibilities do we really have when it comes to the question of health? Without doubt it is part of our nature as living beings that the conscious awareness of health conceals itself. Despite its hidden character, health nonetheless manifests itself in a kind of feeling of well-being. It shows itself above all where such a feeling of well-being means that we are open to new things, ready to embark on new enterprises and, forgetful of ourselves, scarcely

[5] The phenomenological theory of health and illness which is presented below is spelled out in a more complete manner in my study from 2000: *The Hermeneutics of Medicine and the Phenomenology of Health: Steps towards a Philosophy of Medical Practice*, which has recently been published in a revised and updated version (Svenaeus 2022).

> notice the demands and strains which are put upon us. This is what health is (Gadamer 1996: 112, translation altered).

In spite of its character of enigmatic withdrawal, Gadamer consequently sees a possibility of conceptualizing health itself. Unfortunately, he does not provide us with this phenomenological theory of health in his book. What he does give us are some ingenious, albeit unsystematized, hints concerning how we should look upon the phenomenon:

> Health is not a condition that one introspectively feels in oneself. Rather it is a condition of being-there, of being-in-the-world, of being-together-with-other-people, of being taken in by an active and rewarding engagement with the things that matters in life. . . . It is the rhythm of life, a permanent process in which equilibrium re-establishes itself. This is something known to us all. Think of the processes of breathing, digesting, and sleeping for example (Gadamer 1996: 113, translation altered).

The terms that Gadamer uses to characterize health in the quotation – "being-there", "being-in-the-world", "being-with-people", "to be busy with projects in life" – indicate that health is something we live *through* rather than *towards*.[6] As we will see, Gadamer's terminology here is inherited from Heidegger. Illness is obviously an obstruction to health and its transparency; everything that goes on without us paying explicit attention to it when we are healthy – walking, thinking, talking – now offers resistance. The ways of the body, our thinking, the whole world, everything is now "out of tune," coloured by feelings of pain, weakness, and helplessness, like in the case of Toombs' falling ill with MS mentioned above.

5.5 Heidegger's Phenomenology

One obvious shortcoming in Husserl's philosophy – which is Toombs' major source of inspiration – is the absence of a phenomenology of feelings for describing the structure of perceptions, actions and thoughts in the life of an ill person. The "attunement" of the self in its "being-in-the-world" is vital for the understanding of health and illness, and this terminology descends from Heidegger rather than from Husserl. Heidegger, in his main work *Being and Time* (1996), significantly widened the domains of phenomenology. Husserl was mainly concerned with epistemology – the theory of knowledge, with an emphasis on the theory of science; whereas Heidegger rather focused the everyday world of being and understanding. His phenomenology is accordingly what he calls a "fundamental ontology" – investigating different modes of what it means to be, rather than what it means to know.

The "being-in-the-world," the "worldliness" of human persons, is conceptualized by Heidegger by stressing several different aspects of this process. Since the

[6] The hyphens indicate that human beings and the world are thought as a unity and not as subjects and objects. The world is not something external to, but is constitutive for the mode of being of persons.

aspects belong to the only creatures that truly exists, human beings, and not to things, they are called "existentials". Human beings *exist*: that is, they have a relation to their own being, and they are open to the world as a possibility for themselves. This openness to the world is a pattern not only of action, but also of thinking, feeling, and talking. The three important existentials which Heidegger names in *Being and Time* are "understanding," "attunement," and "discourse". These three existentials are thought of as intertwined; they always work together, inseparably, as an attuned, articulated understanding situated in the world. The choice of understanding instead of cognition makes a relation to action possible. Understanding can include the active and incarnated sides of human life; and so can the concepts of attunement and discourse.

To the existence of human beings also belongs an aspect that has not yet reached, and perhaps never will reach, an articulated understanding. This is the territory of feelings. With the aid of Heidegger, it is possible to see how feelings are one aspect of our way of giving meaning to phenomena when we act, think, and speak in the world. Our grasping of a phenomenon is a part of the ongoing, living activity in the world that Heidegger refers to as understanding. But the understanding must always be *attuned* in order to be meaningful: "Every understanding has its mood. Every attunement understands" (1996: 309). Heidegger thus gives feelings, primarily in the form of moods, an important function and position in his philosophy. Moods open up the world to human beings in a precognitive way: "*Mood has always already disclosed being-in-the-world as a whole and first makes possible directing oneself toward something*" (1996: 129, italics in original). We find ourselves already present into the world as attuned (in some type of mood), and these moods are the primary and unarticulated form of being concerned through which we can accommodate ourselves in the meaning-structures of the world.

Attunement cannot simply be equated with different feelings as they are studied by the psychologist. Psychology is what Heidegger refers to as an *ontic* science; it studies the mental states of subjects. Heidegger's fundamental ontology – like Husserl's phenomenology – is developed in order to provide a ground for every such ontic science – psychology as well as biology. Moods form the way we understand and articulate the phenomena in the world, and also, ultimately, the way we understand ourselves and other persons. Things in the world matter to human beings because they are part of a totality of relevance – a cultural tradition – and this "mattering to" is attuned, it feels in a certain way. Certain moods are indeed the prerequisite for reaching what Heidegger calls an *authentic* understanding (1996: 172).

5.6 Homelike Versus Unhomelike Being-in-the-World

Back to the phenomenology of health and illness. Heidegger never wrote anything substantial about the subject. There is no analysis of the structures of the healthy versus the ill existence in *Being and Time*. Although a whole chapter in the second division of the book is devoted to an analysis of the meaning of death, Heidegger never links his ontological interpretation of death as the finitude of human existence to an analysis of the meaning of illness. He makes clear that the existential interpretation of death is prior to any biology or ontology of life, but he also mentions that the medical and biological inquiry into life and dying could be of importance in the analysis of the meaning-structure of human existence (Heidegger 1996: 229). The relation between biology and phenomenology is not further discussed, however, nor is a phenomenology of health and illness developed in the book (or in other books by Heidegger).

It is tempting to interpret the opposition of authenticity and inauthenticity in Heidegger's philosophy as a difference between health and illness, at least when one considers mental health or the "health" of a culture; and some philosophers inspired by Heidegger and Nietzsche have done so (Boss 1979; Welsh 2016). But this is not really an attractive option, at least not if one intends to preserve the normal, everyday meanings of the terms "healthy" and "ill". Authenticity and inauthenticity in Heidegger's phenomenology are two different modes of understanding. These are the counterparts to Husserl's two different modes of attention: the phenomenological attitude and the natural attitude to life.

However, the authentic, philosophical understanding – which in *Being and Time* is reached in the moment of anxiety – would obviously not always be identical with a healthy being-in-the-world (Heidegger 1996: 177). The phenomenologist could be temporarily ill, but still have an authentic understanding, or she could indeed reach it while (or even through) being ill. Also, the phenomenologist would indeed always have to return to the inauthentic understanding of her daily life, since it provides the necessary background for philosophical reflection, by being precisely that which is thereby explored as a pattern of meaning. It would therefore be rather strange to regard every human being living in an inauthentic mood of understanding as ill. In *Being and Time* Heidegger associates the term "the they" with a certain form of everyday existence lacking genuine selfhood and reflection (1996: 118); but though there is certainly some contempt in Heidegger's description of modern public life, he did not mean to suggest that all human beings who never reach authentic understanding are ill.

Despite the shortcomings of the attempts to identify health with authentic existence, it will be instructive here to go back to the account Heidegger gives of existential anxiety in *Being and Time*:

> In anxiety one has an "uncanny" feeling. Here the peculiar indefiniteness of that which Dasein (human being) finds itself involved in with anxiety initially finds expression: the nothing and nowhere. But uncanniness means at the same time a not-being-at-home. In our first phenomenal indication of the fundamental constitution of Dasein (human being) and the clarification of the existential meaning of being-in in contradistinction to the categorical signification of "insideness", being-in was defined as dwelling with . . . , being familiar with . . . (1996, p. 176, my additions in parentheses).

What authentic anxiety makes evident is essentially the same phenomenon that is brought to attention, not in healthy, but in *ill* forms of life – the *not* being at home in the world. Unhomelikeness[7] – which is taken to an extreme in the authentic mood, is, also in our everyday modes of being-in-the-world, a basic aspect of our existence; but there it is hidden by a dominating being *at home* in the world and is therefore covered up (Heidegger 1996: 256).

The being-at-home of human being-there – "dwelling with, being familiar with" – is consequently, at the same time, a being not quite at home in this world. The familiarity of our lifeworld – the world of human actions, projects, and communication – is always also pervaded by a homelessness: this is my world but at the same time I do not fully know it or control it. I will return to this alien nature of the world shortly in discussing illness and the body, a theme that is central to the complementary health and illness approach mentioned above: the tradition proceeding from Merleau-Ponty (Carel 2008; Leder 1990).

Health, in this Heideggerian spirit, is consequently to be understood as a being at home that keeps the not being at home in the world from becoming apparent. The not being at home, which is a basic and necessary condition of human existence, related to our finitude and dependence upon others, is, in illness, brought to attention and transformed into a pervasive homelessness. One of two *a priori* structures of existence – not being at home and being at home – wins out over the other: unhomelikeness takes control of our being-in-the-world. The basic alienness of my being-in-the-world, which in health is always in the process of receding into the background, breaks forth in illness to pervade existence (Svenaeus 2022: Chaps. 2 and 3).

5.7 Attunement and Balance

The *attunement* of our lives consequently is the phenomenon to focus upon, when trying to get hold of the difference between healthy and ill ways of being-in-the-world. To be healthy or ill is, however, certainly not identical with just having a good or a bad feeling. As pointed out, attunement is not the quality of a thing – of an isolated human subject – but rather a being delivered to the world, a finding oneself in the meaning-patterns of the world while engaged in activities. Recall the quotation from Gadamer I gave above:

> Health is not a condition that one introspectively feels in oneself. Rather it is a condition of being-there, of being-in-the-world, of being-together-with-other-people, of being taken in by an active and rewarding engagement with the things that matters in life. . . . It is the rhythm of life, a permanent process in which equilibrium re-establishes itself (Gadamer 1996: 113, translation altered).

[7] The double meaning of the German word "unheimlich" – it means both "uncanny" and "unhomelike" ('unheimisch') – cannot be translated directly into English. For the etymology of the word "unheimlich" and the relation between the phenomenon of *Unheimlichkeit* and mental illness, see Freud (1925); and Trigg (2014).

We now recognize Gadamer's terms as derived from the phenomenology of *Being and Time*, and we are able to understand this healthy, rhythmic being-in-the-world as a form of attunement, which is certainly not a state that one feels in oneself, but which nevertheless has a "tune," a feeling component to it.

Citing another passage from Gadamer's book, I pointed out that the phenomenon of illness appears to be easier to get hold of than the phenomenon of health. When we are healthy everything "flows," the mood we find ourselves in does not make itself heard or seen. It could possibly be felt as a certain form of rhythm in our being-in-the-world connected to time and to the way we are incarnated – to our breathing and to the beating of our hearts. It should not, however, be confused with other *positive* moods like well-being or happiness. Such moods also colour our understanding, but in a much more obvious and manifest way than health does. Health is rather a non-apparent attunement, a rhythmic, balancing mood that supports our understanding in a homelike way without calling for our attention.

The homelikeness of health can in this case not be a balance between two (or several) entities (like in homeostatic health theory). The "balance of health" must phenomenologically refer to the way persons find their place in the world as a meaning pattern – a being-*in*-the-world. Health is thus not a question of a passive state but rather of an active process – a *balancing*. As an illuminating comparative example in exploring balance and its relation to health, we will therefore choose a human activity, namely the everyday activity of riding a bicycle.

The healthy mood – the healthy attuned understanding – is always in the process of receding, since it is a mood of homelikeness. In the same way as you do not think of your homelike being-in-the-world when you are healthy, you do not think of your physical balance when you are riding a bicycle. These moods are similar in this respect, though the first one is more complex, since it is not only an attunement of one activity (bicycling), but of one's entire being-in-the-world. Both are, however, unobtrusive *attunements*, supporting our action and understanding.

If you fall off the bicycle or get ill, however, you will notice. When your balance is challenged – when you ride over a stone, for example – you will make efforts to regain your balance in order not to fall down, but eventually will not succeed and will fall over. The moods of illness, in contrast to healthy attunement, seem to manifest themselves in obtrusive ways, colouring our whole existence and understanding. This is not always an immediate experience – like falling down from a bicycle – but sometimes a gradual process, during which, however, in the same way as in the example of riding a bicycle, one strives constantly to "stay upright," to keep one's balance, but finally has to give in to illness, as in the examples offered by Toombs of MS and other gradually appearing chronic illnesses, such as diabetes (1992).

5.8 The Lived Body and the Broken Tool

Authentic anxiety as Heidegger envisages it in *Being and Time* bears resemblance to the unhomelike attunement of illness, which we have focused on above. The unhomelike attunement of the ill existence would, in contrast to the attunement of authenticity, be relatively long lasting (depending upon being curable or not). It could, however, in a similar way to authentic attunement, in some cases, offer new perspectives on the worldliness of human being.

Certainly not every breakdown in the ongoing activity of being-in-the-world is equivalent to what is experienced in existential anxiety and similarly unhomelike in character. Heidegger's famous example of a limited disruption in *Being and Time* is the broken hammer (1996: 65). While engaged in building a house, we do not, in the act of hammering, explicitly focus our attention upon the hammer in an intentional way. We are absorbed in the activity. Suddenly, the head of the hammer flies off, and the tool can no longer be used for striking nails. The activity is now interrupted, and we are forced to focus upon the hammer, to become conscious of it as a broken tool which must be repaired or replaced, if we are to be able to go on building the house.

Heidegger's point here is that through breakdowns in the activity, it becomes possible to grasp the hammer as a piece of equipment – a tool – and not just as a thing (1996: 68). Similar to authentic understanding, certain breakdowns of activity (which, of course, must also be attuned but not necessarily in the mood of anxiety) make it possible to explicate *parts* of the world-structure as tools. That is, the meaning of the hammer is not revealed if we study it separately as a physical thing with certain qualities – blackness, heaviness, a certain shape and so on – but rather it must be placed in the context of the world as a meaning-structure for human beings.

Heidegger in *Being and Time* neglects to highlight the part played by the body in activity and understanding. He never extensively discusses the body as a set of tools or part of the meaning-structure of the world (Aho 2009; Leder 1990: 83–84). There is no valid argument, however, for restricting the concept of tool as it is used in *Being and Time* to things outside the human body. To place the limit of the meaning-patterns of the world at the surface of the biological organism would be to proceed from a third-person perspective, and not from the phenomenological point of view which Heidegger adopts in this work. Once the positions of dualism and reductionism have been given up in the phenomenological attitude they cannot be brought in again in order to draw a line between the hammer and the hand in the phenomenological analysis. If the hammer and not the hand can be said to constitute a tool in the phenomenological sense, this line of demarcation must be drawn from the phenomenological position.

If the hand instead of the hammer breaks, the activity will likewise come to an end. The hand consequently is also a sort of tool for activity and understanding constituting a nodal point in the meaning-pattern of the world. The hand, like the hammer, can be repaired or maybe even replaced by a prosthesis that would adequately perform the functions of a hand. But the situation of the broken hand is also different from the situation of the broken hammer since it is very differently attuned.

The confusion and annoyance of the broken hammer can hardly be compared to the *pain* we experience when having broken the wrist.[8]

The hand and the hammer are therefore rightly regarded as different forms of tools; but the line of demarcation cannot be drawn with reference to the surface of the biological organism. It is rather determined through an appeal to the importance the tool plays in the totality of relevance for the human being in question. If the tool belongs to the region we would identify with the self rather than the world in the person's being-in-the-world, then it would consequently be more likely to result in illness if broken. The lived body would, in any case, just like language, form a vital part of our transcendence into the world. It would indeed seem appropriate to accord the lived body the status of being the fourth major existential of our being-in-the-world, alongside the understanding, attunement and language in Heidegger's conceptual apparatus. As Merleau-Ponty writes, the body "understands" and "inhabits" the world (2012: 139–148). Illness would mean an unhomelikeness of this structure of being-in, which can be thematized as a peculiar kind of attunement, as a failure in transcendence, or as a breakdown in the tool-structure related to the self.

Richard Zaner in *The Context of Self* investigates different ways in which the body announces itself as uncanny in illness (1981: 48–55). This book is an early classic in English speaking medical phenomenology and an important source of inspiration for Toombs (and myself). My body is not just a tool that I use or a dwelling I live in (this is the basic mistake of dualism) – it is *me* (failing to recognize the significance of this "mineness" is the basic mistake of reductionism). I *am* my own body. Yet this body, as Zaner remarks, also has a life of its own. As we have come to realize through our reading of Heidegger, I belong to the world just as much as the world belongs to me. In the same way I also belong to my body:

> If there is a sense in which my own-body is "intimately mine," there is furthermore, an equally decisive sense in which I belong to it – in which I am at its disposal or mercy, if you will. My body, like the world in which I live, has its own nature, functions, structures, and biological conditions; since it embodies me, I thus experience myself as implicated by my body and these various conditions, functions, etc. I am exposed to whatever can influence, threaten, inhibit, alter, or benefit my biological organism. Under certain conditions, it can fail me (more or less), not be capable of fulfilling my wants or desires, or even thoughts, forcing me to turn away from what I may want to do and attend to my own body: because of fatigue, hunger, thirst, disease, injury, pain, or even itches, I am forced at times to tend and attend to it, regardless, it may be, of what may well seem more urgent at the moment (Zaner 1981: 52).

The body is an alien, yet, at the same time, myself. It involves biological processes beyond my control, but these processes still belong to me as lived by me. The body seems to be the very form of finitude, in the sense of referring to our being born as well as our having to die. Illness is an uncanny and unhomelike experience since the otherness of the body then presents itself in an obtrusive, merciless way. The behavior of the body in illness is often no longer under the person's full control. It refuses

[8] For a survey and critical discussion of the different characterizations and theories of pain found in the phenomenological tradition, see Svenaeus (2020).

to obey the wishes of the ill person – when she becomes unable to move around in the way typical for healthy being-in-the-world. And the emptying of bowel and bladder may take place without the ill person being able to regulate it.

Of course, the body has a life of its own even in health – certain needs must be satisfied; but the inconvenience, experienced in health, of urgently having to heed the call of nature, is very different from the inconvenience of urinating or defecating without noticing it until it is too late. The change in outer appearance and the loss of mastery over one's own body, which take place in many cases of illness, can in themselves be stigmatizing and lead to problems in the relationship with other people, which is an important theme in the study by Toombs presented above 1992: Chap. 4).

5.9 Conclusion

The phenomenological focus upon health and illness, as aspects of our embodied being-in-the-world, is intended to form, not an alternative, but rather a complement to a biomedical science of diseases. Doctors and other medical professionals are indeed very interested in diseases in attempting to heal patients and for very good reasons. What the phenomenologists criticize are a too narrow approach to the goal of clinical practice and not biomedical science itself. Given that the goal of the clinical encounter is to restore lost health, the biomedical image of health – absence of diseases – would tend to make medicine identical with applied biology. But this is neither what medicine is or what it ought to be. Medicine is a meeting between two persons and an interpretation of the ill person's being-in-the-world, with the aim of restoring a life that has turned unhomelike. To find diseases and to cure or mitigate them form significant parts of this activity, but the activity includes much more than that.

The point of phenomenological approaches to medicine is to give a general characteristic of health and illness and provide a vocabulary with the aid of which one can talk about different illnesses and different ill persons and, in each case, be able to understand why and how *this* person is ill. However, this does not mean that all phenomenology can give us is good descriptions of what different individuals experience. The phenomenological description aims at uncovering necessary features of the meaning-patterns structuring our life. What breaks down in illness are precisely the meaning-patterns of being-*in*-the-world, the way we inhabit the world through our attuned, understanding activities. The unhomelikeness of illness is consequently a certain form of senselessness, an attunement of, for instance, disorientedness, helplessness, resistance, and despair. To understand this predicament and find ways of making life less unhomelike for ill persons is the mission of health-care practitioners. Clinical empathy, illness stories and person-centred approaches to the patient's suffering – Toombs' signposts – are still feasible roads forwards in this domain, but they should be anchored in a phenomenological understanding of the "healing relationship" (Toombs 1992: 110).

References

Aho, Kevin. 2009. *Heidegger's Neglect of the Body*. New York: SUNY.
Aho, Kevin, ed. 2018. *Existential Medicine: Essays on Health and Illness*. Rowman & Littlefield.
Aho, James, and Kevin Aho. 2008. *Body Matters: A Phenomenology of Sickness, Disease, and Illness*. Lanham, MD: Lexington Books.
Boss, Medard. 1979. *Existential Foundations of Medicine and Psychology*. Trans. S. Convay and A. Cleaves. Jason Aronson Publisher.
Carel, Havi. 2008. *Illness: The Cry of the Flesh*. Acumen Publishing.
Carel, Havi. 2016. *Phenomenology of Illness*. Oxford University Press.
Cassell, Eric J. 1991. *The Nature of Suffering*. Oxford University Press.
Charon, Rita. 2006. *Narrative Medicine: Honoring the Stories of Illness*. Oxford University Press.
Decety, Jean, ed. 2012. *Empathy: From Bench to Bedside*. MIT Press.
Freud, Sigmund. 1925. The Uncanny. In *Collected Papers*, vol. 4. (trans: A. Strachey), 368–407. The Hogarth Press.
Gadamer, Hans-Georg, 1996. *The Enigma of Health: The Art of Healing in a Scientific Age*. Trans. J. Gaiger and N. Walker. Stanford University Press.
Gallagher, Shaun. 2005. *How the Body Shapes the Mind*. Oxford University Press.
Heidegger, Martin. 1996. *Being and Time*. Trans. J. Stambaugh. State University of New York Press.
Jonas, Hans. 1984. *The Imperative of Responsibility: In Search of Ethics for the Technological Age*. University of ChicagoPress.
Leder, Drew. 1990. *The Absent Body*. University of Chicago Press.
Leder, Drew. 1992. *The Body in Medical Thought and Practice (no. 43)*. Kluwer.
Leder, Drew. 2016. *The Distressed Body: Rethinking Illness, Imprisonment, and Healing*. University of Chicago Press.
Leder, Drew. 2024. *The Healing Body: Creative Responses to Illness, Aging and Affliction*. Northwestern University Press.
Marcum, James A. 2017. Patient- and Person-Centered Medicine: Does the Center Hold? *In The Bloomsbury Companion to Contemporary Philosophy of Medicine*, ed. J. A. Marcum. London: Bloomsbury, pp. 249–274.
Merleau-Ponty, Maurice. 2012. *Phenomenology of Perception*. (trans: Landes, D. A.). Routledge.
Ratcliffe, Matthew. 2008. *Feelings of Being: Phenomenology, Psychiatry and the Sense of Reality*. Oxford University Press.
Slatman, Jenny. 2014. *Our Strange Body: Philosophical Reflections on Identity and Medical Interventions*. Amsterdam University Press.
Spicker, Stuart F., ed. 1978. *Organism, Medicine and Metaphysics. Essays in Honor of Hans Jonas on his 75th Birthday*. Vol. no. 7. Kluwer.
Svenaeus, Fredrik. 2009. The Phenomenology of Falling Ill: An Explication, Critique and Improvement of Sartre's Theory of Embodiment and Alienation. *Human Studies* 32 (1): 53–66.
Svenaeus, Fredrik. 2017. *Phenomenological Bioethics: Medical Technologies, Human Suffering, and the Meaning of Being Alive*. Routledge.
Svenaeus, Fredrik. 2020. *Pain, in Routledge Handbook of Phenomenology of Emotions*. Eds. T. Szanto and H. Landweer. London: Routledge, pp. 543–552.
Svenaeus, Fredrik. 2022. *The Hermeneutics of Medicine and the Phenomenology of Health: Steps Towards a Philosophy of Medical Practice*. second revised edition. Springer.
Toombs, S. Kay. 1992. *The Meaning of Illness: A Phenomenological Account of the Different Perspectives of Physician and Patient*. Vol. no. 42. Kluwer.
Toombs, S. Kay, ed. 2001. *Handbook of Phenomenology and Medicine*. Vol. no. 68. Kluwer.
Trigg, Dylan. 2014. *The Thing: A Phenomenology of Horror*. Zero Books.
Welsh, Talia. 2016. Many Healths: Nietzsche and Phenomenologies of Illness. *Frontiers of Philosophy in China* 11 (3): 338–357.
Zaner, Richard M. 1981. *The Context of Self: A Phenomenological Inquiry Using Medicine as a Clue*. Ohio University Press.
Zaner, Richard M., ed. 1988. *Death: Beyond Whole-Brain Criteria (no. 31)*. Kluwer.

Chapter 6
Does the Philosophy of Medicine Exist: A Reappraisal

Søren Holm

6.1 Introduction

In 1992 Arthur Caplan published a paper arguing that the philosophy of medicine did not exist as a field of inquiry. He summarized his argument as follows:

> In order to constitute a field, an inquiry must be well-integrated with other cognate inquiries and disciplines, have an established canon of key books, textbooks, anthologies and articles, and a set of distinctive and defining problems. The philosophy of medicine as it currently exists fails to satisfy these criteria and, thus, fails to exist as a field of inquiry.

Caplan lamented the non-existence of the philosophy of medicine as a field of inquiry since many of the discussion in medical ethics/bioethics rely on contested concepts foundation to medical research and practice that need analysis. He also acknowledged that although there is no 'philosophy **of** medicine', there is considerable scholarly activity that can be described correctly as 'philosophy **and** medicine'. Philosophy & Medicine is also the name of the book series in which this chapter is published, and which I co-edit. The question raised by Caplan in the title of his paper, a title which I have partly re-used for this chapter, can in the context of the book series be reformulated to: (1) Has Philosophy & Medicine ever published any 'philosophy of medicine', and if so (2) does Philosophy & Medicine constitute part of the canon of 'philosophy of medicine'?

In this chapter I will argue that Caplan's conclusion is wrong. That is, I will argue that there is a field of inquiry which can properly be denoted as 'philosophy **of**

S. Holm (✉)
Centre for Social Ethics and Policy, University of Manchester, Manchester, UK

Center for Medical Ethics, HELSAM, University of Oslo, Oslo, Norway
e-mail: soren.holm@manchester.ac.uk

L. M. Rasmussen, S. Holm (eds.), *50 Years of Philosophy and Medicine*, Philosophy and Medicine 150, https://doi.org/10.1007/978-3-031-95175-6_6

medicine'.[1] I will first present Caplan's argument in more detail and elucidate and criticise some of the key assumptions and stipulations that he makes. I will then show that philosophy of medicine does have an established canon and a set of distinctive and defining problems, and that it engages appropriately with other cognate inquiries and disciplines. Caplan's analyses and claim of the non-existence of philosophy of medicine was already critiqued immediately following the publication of the 1992 paper, and I will build on and extend that critique (Wulff 1992; Velanovich 1994; Pellegrino 1998). I believe, but will not argue directly for the view that Caplan's conclusion was already unwarranted in 1992, which co-incidentally is the year I started my PhD studies at 'Afdeling for medicinsk videnskabsteori',[2] at the University of Copenhagen.

Some may take the argument in this chapter to be superfluous, since the existence of philosophy of medicine is now much more generally accepted. There is a Stanford Encyclopedia of Philosophy entry for 'Philosophy of Medicine' claiming in direct response to Caplan that:

> … as there are now dedicated journals and professional organizations, a relatively well-established canon of scholarly literature, and distinctive questions and problems, it is defensible to claim that philosophy of medicine has now established itself.

And there is a two volume 'Handbook of the Philosophy of Medicine' published by Springer, with 68 chapters of which Caplan himself has authored one on the topic of "How Can Aging Be Thought of as Anything Other Than a Disease?" (Schramme and Edwards 2017; Caplan 2017)

I nevertheless think that a re-evaluation of Caplan's arguments is appropriate since philosophy of medicine, if it exists, is always at risk of being amalgamated into and subsumed by one of the larger adjoining fields of inquiry, e.g. bioethics, medical humanities, or science and technology studies. A better understanding of the mode of existence of philosophy of medicine might therefore be useful in order to delimit the field more precisely.

There is an interesting question about the relationship between medical ethics/bioethics and philosophy of medicine. Medical ethics is clearly a philosophical engagement with important aspects of medicine, including both medical research and medical practices, and it is probably best described as a particular sub-field of practical moral philosophy (Bennett et al. 2002). It could therefore, without contradiction be seen as a part of philosophy of medicine. If medical ethics/bioethics was seen as a part of philosophy of medicine Caplan's worries about integration, canon, and distinctive and defining problems would presumably be alleviated, since at least the largest sub-field of philosophy of medicine would then fulfil the Caplan criteria to a reasonable degree. We might still have concerns about integration with the most recent developments in moral philosophy or about the quality of the canon, but there would undoubtedly be both some integration and a canon. We might also have the kind of concerns raised by Henk ten Have and William Stempsey among many others that medical ethics activity is displacing all other activities in the philosophy of medicine (ten Have 1997; Stempsey 2007).

[1] I will from here on drop the quotation marks, unless required by the context.

[2] Literal translation 'Section for theory of medical science'.

In this chapter I will accept Caplan's view that medical ethics/bioethics is not part of the philosophy of medicine proper, although his argument for this position is not very convincing. Caplan argues rightly that analysis of moral and legal issues is different from analysis of logic, methods and conceptual foundations (Caplan 1992). But, this only shows that medical ethics/bioethics falls outside of philosophy of medicine, if we have already decided by stipulation that philosophy of medicine is about the latter set of questions, only. In this chapter I also accept Caplan's view that medical humanities is a separate field, although again there is an interesting question about the position of the philosophical aesthetics of medicine.

6.2 Caplan's Argument Further Explicated

The existence of the philosophy of medicine as a field is plausibly an ontological question (Caplan 1992, p. 68), but it is clearly a question about social ontology. Academic or scholarly fields do not exist and are not classified as natural kinds. They come into and go out of existence through complex social processes. Some parts of philosophy and what we now recognise as the field of psychology were, for instance once united in the field of natural philosophy, but are now completely distinct fields. As William Stempsey points out:

> How a discipline is delineated is often largely a question of pragmatic usefulness rather than any reflection of fundamental ontological realities. (Stempsey 2004, p. 247)

In the section "What is a field?" in his paper Caplan provides a more extended account of the three criteria mentioned above, i.e. integration, canon, and distinctive and defining problems.

In relation to integration he argues that philosophy of medicine "is not well integrated with the rest of either philosophy or medicine" and that only few philosophers and few doctors know or are aware of the work in philosophy of medicine (Caplan 1992, p. 72). He therefore describes philosophy of medicine as "an intellectual island". In relation to the canon he writes that "fields in the humanities must have a paradigmatic or exemplary core" (Caplan 1992, p. 73) and that a reliable test of the existence of such a canonical core is "whether or not disputes rage about the composition of the canon". Finally he identifies key, defining puzzles in the philosophy of biology and argues that in comparison philosophy of medicine has only a few defining problems, before claiming that there is actually only one real contender for a defining problem, namely "the debate about the meaning of the concepts of 'health' and 'disease'" (Caplan 1992, p. 73).

In the following I will first analyse whether philosophy of medicine has a core set of defining problems, then move on to the existence of a canon, and finally investigate the issue of integration with cognate fields.

6.3 The Core Areas of Inquiry

Does philosophy of medicine have core areas of inquiry or problems that are distinctive and definitive for the field? In their article in the Stanford Encyclopedia of Philosophy Reiss and Ankeny identify 12 core debates in the field:

1. "How Should We Define Health and Disease?
2. Contested and Controversial Disease Categories
3. Theories, Causes, and Explanations in Medicine
4. Reductionism and Holism in Medicine
5. Randomized Controlled Trials and Evidence-Based Medicine
6. Animal Models
7. Observational Studies and Case Reports
8. Diagnosis
9. Clinician Judgement and the Role of Expertise
10. How Are Collective Expert Judgments Made in Medicine?
11. Values in Medical Research
12. Measuring Medical Outcomes" (Reiss and Ankeny 2022, original publication date 2016)

This listing is, however not exhaustive and may be skewed towards issues where philosophy of medicine interacts with philosophy of science. We should as a minimum add three other core issues to the list: the philosophical phenomenology of health and illness, the analysis of the meaning of suffering, and the question of whether medicine has a set of internal goals (and what they are). For each of these additions there is both an active research literature, a canon, and important links to philosophy in general.

The prominence of each core topic in the overall panorama of the philosophy of medicine vaxes and vanes over time, and some topics may eventually be passed on to other fields in whole or in part, as has happened to some degree with the study of clinical decision-making. Some of the core topics are also core in other fields. If we for instance conceptualise a three circle Venn diagram between philosophy of medicine, philosophy of psychiatry,[3] and philosophy of psychology there will be very considerable overlaps in core topics of inquiry, although each field may have its own inflection in how a topic is analysed and discussed.

The precise delineation of distinctive and definining issues depend on whether we take a narrow or a broad view on the scope and limits of the field (Stempsey 2004). Some argue that the proper scope of philosophy **of** medicine is narrow, and that it has to be distinguished from other activities that also involve an interaction between philosophy and medicine. Edmund Pellegrino and David Thomasma for instance distinguishes philosoph of medicine from philosophy **and** medicine, and philosophy **in** medicine (Pellegrino and Thomasma 1981). Philosophy and

[3] For the moment bracketing the issue of whether philosophy of psychiatry is a field in itself, or a sub-field of philosophy of medicine.

medicine concerns itself with problems that both areas of inquiry share, but each contributes its own distinctive input and the inquiries are not integrated but proceed on parallel tracks. Philosophy in medicine is the application of the tools of philosophy to a medical problem, including problems in the medical sciences. Finally, philosophy of medicine is the field providing philosophical analysis of the conceptual foundations of clinical medical practice, only. Its scope is exclusively those phenomena that are "peculiar to the human encounter with health, illness, disease, death, and the desire for prevention and healing" (Pellegrino 1998, p. 327). On this narrow conception many of the items listed on Reiss and Ankeny's list, e.g. 'Randomized controlled trials and evidence-based medicine' or 'Animal models', would fall outside of the scope of philosophy of medicine.

A broad view of the scope of philosophy of medicine includes philosophical analyses of the scientific basis of medicine and the practices of medical scientists, as well as analyses of clinical medical practice. That is, it includes the field of philosophy in medicine as defined by Pellegrino and Thomasma within the philosophy of medicine (Stempsey 2004). The broad view is also much less prescriptive *a priori*. We can't necessarily decide in advance whether or not a philosophical analysis of a particular question is within or outside the scope of philosophy of medicine. That may to some extent depend on whether the analysis actually illuminates or explicates an issue in medicine, or whether the analysis primarily uses a medical example to illuminate or explicate an issue in philosophy. There are many reasons to prefer the broad view of the scope of philosophy of medicine. First, it is congruent with the self-understanding of most of the people working in the field, e.g. in relation to analysis of issues peculiar to the medical sciences or peculiar to evidence based medicine. Most philosophers of medicine would accept those areas as part of the core of the field, even if it is not the areas they themselves work in (Stempsey 2008). Second, a stipulation that the field is limited to the analysis of phenomena "peculiar to the human encounter with…" also seems to restrictive. In relation to an analysis of the concepts of health and disease there must be a question about whether these concepts have general scope across all or a sub-class of biological organisms, or whether restricted in some way to humans, and answering that question again seems to fall within the core of philosophy of medicine. Philosophy of medicine is not identical to philosophy of biology, but the overlapping areas of interests between these two fields should not be excluded from one of them by stipulation.

6.4 The Canon

Is there an established canon of key works in the philosophy of medicine? A quick, but perhaps slightly facetious answer is again to point to Reiss and Ankeny's encyclopedia entry. For each of the 12 core debates they identify, they also identify the papers or books that are today seen as initiating the debate, and a raft of later papers clarifying, criticising, extending etc. the analysis and conclusions provided in the early works. This looks very much what one would expect to find if there is a canon that is recognised and forms the basis for further work in the field.

An even quicker way it to ask ChatGPT to identify the 10 most important books in the philosophy of medicine, which it is happy to do with the claim that "These texts provide a solid foundation for exploring the philosophical dimensions of medicine, touching on ethics, epistemology, and the nature of illness and healing" (Fig. 6.1). Unfortunately, a perusal of the list produced shows that some of the details provided are examples of large language model hallucinations, and that the list is therefore unreliable.

More seriously, it is, in fact relatively easy to identify key early works that are still cited in and seen as central to discussions of the core areas of inquiry. Some of these are identified in relation to the concepts of health, illness, and disease in the contributions by Bjørn Hofmann and Mary Ann Cutter to this volume, and others in the contribution by Fredrik Svenaeus on the phenomenology of health and illness. There are also many examples in the literature where explicit claims are made about canonical status of a particular work or body of work. Here it should suffice to quote one to establish that there is a recognised canon from the internal perspective of those engaged in philosophy of medicine. In an introduction to a symposium on Christopher Boorse's work Thomas Schramme writes:

> Similarly to what Robert Nozick once said about John Rawls's work, it can be demanded that philosophers of medicine must now either work within Boorse's theory or explain why not. It is simply the main contender in the so-called naturalist camp of contributions to the theory of disease (Schramme 2014, p. 565)

There are a number of recognised core journals in the field. All of these publish work on philosophy of medicine, as well as work on medical ethics, but they are clearly distinguishable from on the one hand journals that publish medical ethics and bioethics work only, and on the other hand journals that publish philosophy of science or science and technology studies across a broader, or the whole spectrum of sciences. Among the core journals in philosophy and medicine are Theoretical Medicine & Bioethics (published since 1979, originally as Theoretical Medicine), the Journal of Medicine and Philosophy (published since 1975), and Medicine, Health Care and Philosophy (the official journal of the European Society for Philosophy of Medicine and Health Care, published since 1997).

The number of relevant and active book series is too large to enumerate but Philosophy & Medicine clearly falls within the category of core book series defining the contours of the field. The series has published works on philosophy of medicine throughout its 50 years of existence. The first volume published in the Philosophy & Medicine series in 1975 was on 'Evaluation and Explanation in the Biomedical Sciences' and one of the books published in 2024 is on 'A Pragmatic Approach to Conceptualization of Health and Disease' (Engelhardt and Spicker 1975; Schermer and Binney 2024). The two editions of the definitive 'Handbook of Analytic Philosophy of Medicine' were also published in Philosophy & Medicine (Sadegh-Zadeh 2015).

In a 2008 paper William Stempsey provided a content analysis of the papers and books published in Theoretical Medicine and Bioethics, the Journal of Medicine and Philosophy, and Philosophy & Medicine between 1997–2006. He found that of

ChatGPT 4o mini – 07.10.2024 ***Reproduced verbatim with uncorrected ChatGPT hallucinations***

You said:
What are the 10 most important books in philosophy of medicine?

ChatGPT said:
The philosophy of medicine explores fundamental questions about health, illness, and the practice of medicine. Here are ten influential books that have shaped this field:

"The Structure of Scientific Revolutions" by Thomas S. Kuhn

Explores how scientific paradigms shift, relevant to understanding changes in medical practices and theories.

"The Philosophy of Medicine: A New Perspective on the Science of Healing" by Harold E.Himmelfarb

Discusses the interplay between medical science and philosophical thought.

"Medical Ethics: A Very Short Introduction" by Tony Hope

Provides an overview of key ethical issues in medicine, blending philosophy with practical implications.

"The Nature of Medical Evidence" by H. K. S. Ashworth

Examines the epistemological aspects of evidence in medicine, including what counts as valid medical evidence.

"The Patient's Ordeal: A Philosopher's Journey Through the Medical Maze" by Eric J. Cassell

Explores the experience of illness from a philosophical standpoint, emphasizing the patient's perspective.

"Philosophy and Medicine" by H. H. J. C. B. S. de Boer

Investigates various philosophical approaches to understanding medicine and health.

"The Body in Pain: The Making and Unmaking of the World" by Elaine Scarry

Analyzes how pain affects perception and understanding, relevant to discussions on illness and medical treatment.

"The Illness Narratives: Suffering, Healing, and the Human Condition" by Arthur W. Frank

Looks at personal narratives of illness, offering insights into the subjective experience of health.

"Thinking About Medicine: From the Perspective of a Philosopher" by H. Tristram Engelhardt Jr.

Delivers a philosophical analysis of medical practices and the moral dilemmas inherent in them.

"On the Medical Humanities" by Michael D. Bayliss

Explores the intersection of medicine and the humanities, emphasizing the importance of a holistic understanding of health.

These texts provide a solid foundation for exploring the philosophical dimensions of medicine, touching on ethics, epistemology, and the nature of illness and healing.

Fig. 6.1 Screenshot of ChatGPT identification of the 10 most important books in philosophy of medicine

the 625 articles analysed 463 had a primary focus on ethics (74%), 162 had a primary focus on the philosophy of medicine (16%) including 110 on metaphysics, 47 on epistemology, 3 on logic, and 2 on aesthetics. Of the 36 books 21 were primarily about ethics (58%), 12 about metaphysics including phenomenology, and 1 about epistemology. The remaining 3 were collections of essays concerned with philosophy of medicine as a field of inquiry (Stempsey 2008). There is thus some empirical evidence for a small, but consistent level of activity in philosophy of medicine published in the core journals and book series of the field.

Given that the philosophy of medicine in its current form is a relatively new field of inquiry with an *a fortiori* relatively new canon it is questionable to what extent we should expect "disputes [to] rage about the composition of the canon". There are many much more established philosophical fields where we do have disputes raging about exclusions from the traditional canon in relation to the importance of historical female contributors to the development of the field, or in relation to decolonisation. It would, however be odd to expect exactly the same kind of disputes in philosophy of medicine where the 'traditional' canon does, for the most part not extend much further back than the 1960s (see for instance the references in Reiss and Ankeny 2022; and for the history of pre-modern philosophy of medicine see King 1978; Löwy 1990). We should of course, expect disputes about the contribution of other voices to the ongoing discourse and work in philosophy of medicine, but that is slightly different than disputes about the canon.

6.5 The Relationship to Cognate Fields

If philosophy of medicine exists it exists in an interplay with other cognate fields. As mentioned above Caplan conceptualises the field as "a sub-discipline of the philosophy of science" (Caplan 1992, p. 69), but that does not seem quite right since 'medicine' as a field is both a field of science and a field of practice. A philosophy of medicine must interrogate medicine both as a science and as a field of practice, and must also interrogate the interaction between the two aspects of medicine. Caplan's characterisation may plausibly be related to his disciplinary background leading him to conceptualise philosophy of medicine, should it exist, as a sub-field of philosophy, and not as a potential sub-field of medicine or a hybrid field relating to more than one parent discipline (Wulff 1992; Stempsey 2004).

Caplan's observation that only few philosophers and few doctors know or are even aware of work in the philosophy of medicine is probably empirically true. It is, however not obvious that it entails that philosophy of medicine is not a *bona fide* field. Only a few philosophers know or are aware of recent work in philosophical logic, e.g. work in modal or temporal logic. They may all have had a compulsory undergraduate course in logic covering the basics of syllogisms, propositional and first order predicate logic, but most have no continued interest in logic and do not read further to understand other logics, and do not follow work in the field. This obviously does not mean that, say temporal logic does not exist as a sub-sub-field of philosophy, or that it is not properly integrated with philosophy as such. For any large, overarching field it will be the case that most people working in the field are ignorant of the work and questions being pursued in most of the sub-fields of their discipline.

Caplan additionally argues that if philosophy of medicine existed, we should expect that:

> … it would and should be the topic of much debate, anguish, posturing and mutual recrimination between those doing the philosophizing and those actual [*sic*] engaged in the daily practice of medicine (Caplan 1992, p. 70).

The warrant for this claim of what we should expect is quite opaque. Most practising scientists are not particularly interested in or anguished by current discussions about evidence, truth, causation, or the social construction of knowledge as discussed in philosophy of science or science and technology studies, and it is difficult to find a reason why those in the medical field should be more interested than scientists in other fields. Scientists and doctors may be vaguely aware of the philosophical debates, but as long as they don't actually influence the practice of science and what is seen within the scientific or practitioner communities as good practice, they are unlikely to spend much energy on debating or posturing.

As Henrik Wulff[4] rightly points out in his response to Caplan medical doctors are a very heterogeneous group with highly variable degrees of interest in any kind of philosophy. Even within the relatively small sub-group of physicians that has an interest in philosophy Wulff further identifies three distinct types, *category 2a* who "are members of the medical profession who have lost interest in the progress of medicine and have taken up philosophy as a hobby, just as some of their colleagues have taken up yachting or golf" (Wulff 1992, p. 80); *category 3a* to which the author of this chapter belongs who "are members of the medical profession who at an early stage after their final exams took up philosophical studies and some of them even have a degree in philosophy" (Wulff 1992, p. 80), and finally category *category 3b* who "are also members of the medical profession (or they belong to one of the other health care professions), They are actively engaged in clinical medicine and do not have sufficient time to immerse themselves in philosophical studies to the same extent as the members of the other categories" (Wulff 1992, p. 80–1).

In most cases it will only be doctors who belong to one of Wulff's three categories who will regularly engage with philosophical work, whether that be work in philosophy of medicine, or (merely?) philosophy and medicine. Members of category 3a or the philosophers working in philosophy of medicine may think and hope that their work should lead to "much debate" and a change in medical practice, but in most cases it will not, even if they can engage and enthuse those in category 2a and 3b. The translational chain between, for instance a fundamental reconceptualization of the concept of disease, and an actual change in disease classification is just too long and too dependent on engaging and enthusing those who are outside of

[4] I have a personal conflict of interest to declare here since Henrik Wulff was my main PhD supervisor.

Wulff's categories of the interested. A very similar point was made by Velanovich already in 1994:

> Why don't practicing physicians care about the philosophy of medicine? Although I do not have hard data to support my opinion, I think there are three possible answers: (1) They are not aware that philosophical issues exist. Or if they are aware, they do not feel that these problems are of practical importance. (2) Many work-a-day physicians do not even keep up with the change of the practical knowledge within their field, let alone theoretical knowledge. (3) Physicians are problem solvers by nature and trade and as such wish to know only that information which will help them solve clinical problems. Traditionally, physicians are intellectual conservatives and view with (at least initial) scepticism edicts from academia that a foundational change in their mode of thinking is warranted. For example, witness the slow conversion to the use of statistical analysis in clinical research and even slower spread of the understanding of statistics among practicing physicians. The increase in the number of physicians understanding the applications of statistical analysis is due more to the teaching of this subject in college and medical school rather than by widespread self-education of extant practicing clinical physicians. I suspect that same will be true of the philosophy of medicine (Velanovich 1994, p. 80).

There are, however some cases where we can point to philosophical work within the philosophy of medicine that has had the effects that Caplan calls for. Sometimes it is because the philosophical work speaks to an issue that is already contentious for other reasons, e.g. at the time of writing questions about the proper conceptualisation of gender diversity and the pharmaceutical treatment of transgender children, adolescents and adults (Giordano 2023). Sometimes it is because those in Wulff's category 3b spot a concept that is practically important but unclear and therefore requires philosophical work, e.g. at the time of writing the concept of 'overdiagnosis' (Hofmann 2014). In both types of cases the philosophical analysis speaks to a current issue that, as an issue is already of interest to medical researchers and practitioners.

6.6 Conclusion

This chapter has argued that philosophy of medicine is a *bona fide* field of research. It may not be a big field, but it has a set of defining problems, a canon of recognised classical works, and an appropriate connection to other cognate fields. Philosophy of medicine may be a small island, but it is not isolated. It has ferries, bridges and tunnels to many other islands in the philosophical archipelago and further afield; and is securely anchored to the continent of medical research and practice. Like most small islands its influence on world affairs is limited, but now and again its voice is heard, and it does make a real impact. The island does not suffer from overpopulation, but it is not experiencing population collapse either; and despite it being yoked to the much larger island of bioethics in the 'philosophy with and for medicine' federation it still manages to maintain its intellectual identity and distinctiveness through the concerted efforts of those keeping its journals, book series and conferences alive and well. As a book series Philosophy & Medicine has played a role in maintaining philosophy of medicine as a vibrant field by publishing high quality work in the field for the last 50 years.

References

Bennett, Rebecca, Charles A. Erin, John Harris, and Søren Holm. 2002. Bioethics, Genethics and Medical Ethics. In *The Blackwell Companion to Philosophy*, 499–516. Blackwell.

Caplan, Arthur L. 1992. Does the Philosophy of Medicine Exist? *Theoretical Medicine* 13:67–77.

Caplan, Arthur. 2017. How Can Aging Be Thought of as Anything Other Than a Disease. In *Handbook of the Philosophy of Medicine*, vol. 1, 233–240. Springer.

Engelhardt Jr, H. Tristram, Stuart Spicker. eds. 1975. Evaluation and Explanation in the Biomedical Sciences. Reidel.

Giordano, Simona. 2023. *Children and Gender: Ethical Issues in Clinical Management of Transgender and Gender Diverse Youth, from Early Years to Late Adolescence*. Oxford University Press.

Hofmann, Bjørn. 2014. Diagnosing Overdiagnosis: Conceptual Challenges and Suggested Solutions. *European Journal of Epidemiology* 29 (9): 599–604.

King, Lester S. 1978. *The Philosophy of Medicine: The Early Eighteenth Century*. Harvard University Press.

Löwy, Ilana. 1990. *The Polish School of Philosophy of Medicine: From Tytus Chalubinski (1820–1889) to Ludwik Fleck (1896–1961)*. Vol. 37. Kluwer.

Pellegrino, Edmund D. 1998. What the Philosophy of Medicine Is. *Theoretical Medicine and Bioethics* 19:315–336.

Pellegrino, Edmund D., and David C. Thomasma. 1981. *A Philosophical Basis of Medical Practice*. Oxford University Press.

Reiss, Julian, and Rachel A. Ankeny. 2022. Philosophy of Medicine. In *The Stanford Encyclopedia of Philosophy*. (Spring 2022 Edition); https://plato.stanford.edu/archives/spr2022/entries/medicine/.

Sadegh-Zadeh, Kazem. 2015. *Handbook of Analytic Philosophy of Medicine*. Vol. 119. Springer. 2012 (1st ed.) & 2015 (2nd ed.).

Schermer, Maartje, Nicholas Binney, eds. 2024. A Pragmatic Approach to Conceptualization of Health and Disease. Springer.

Schramme, Thomas. 2014. Christopher Boorse and the Philosophy of Medicine. *Journal of Medicine and Philosophy* 39 (6): 565–571.

Schramme, Thomas, and Steven Edwards, eds. 2017. *Handbook of the Philosophy of Medicine*. Springer.

Stempsey, William E. 2004. The Philosophy of Medicine: Development of a Discipline. *Medicine, Health Care and Philosophy* 7:243–251.

Stempsey, William E. 2007. Medical Humanities and Philosophy: Is the Universe Expanding or Contracting? *Medicine, Health Care and Philosophy* 10:373–383.

Stempsey, William E. 2008. Philosophy of Medicine Is What Philosophers of Medicine Do. *Perspectives in Biology and Medicine* 51 (3): 379–391.

ten Have, Henk A. M. J. 1997. From Synthesis and System to Morals and Procedure: The Development of Philosophy of Medicine. In *Philosophy and Medicine*, vol. 50, 105–124. Springer.

Velanovich, Vic. 1994. Does the Philosophy of Medicine Exist? A Commentary on Caplan. *Theoretical Medicine* 15:77–81.

Wulff, Henrik R. 1992. Philosophy of Medicine—From a Medical Perspective. *Theoretical Medicine* 13:79–85.

Part II
The Subseries of Philosophy and Medicine

Chapter 7
Volumes on the History of Medical Ethics in the Philosophy and Medicine Series

Robert Baker

The ancient Athenians believed their city was founded by a Greek goddess, Athena, who sprung fully formed from the head of Zeus as a wise and beautiful goddess, armored to defend her city and its citizens. Bioethicists share a similar origin story, believing that their field was founded in a similar fashion, emerging fully formed from the minds of Daniel Callahan, Willard Gaylin, and André Hellegers, wise, good, and armed to defend the rights of patients and research subjects. Since, in both origin tales, their subjects emerged fully formed, neither Athenians nor bioethicists have any reason to probe any prior history. In 1988, I was lunching with two historians of medicine, Dorothy and Roy Porter, when I happened to mention the similarity between Athenians' and bioethicists' origin stories. My historian friends immediately suggested that we challenge bioethicists' origin "myth" by bringing historians and bioethicists together to explore precursors to bioethics.

To implement this idea the three of us drafted a proposal to the Wellcome Institute requesting funding for a pair of conferences on the historical development of medical ethics in Britain and America. The Institute funded our proposal, and we brought together eleven historians of medicine, (Peter Bartrip, Chester Burns, M. Anne Crowther, Mary Fissell, Johanna Geyer-Kordesch, David Harley, John Pickstone, Dorothy Porter, Roy Porter, Stanley J. Reiser, and Russell G. Smith), and four bioethicists trained in philosophy, Tom Beauchamp, Laurence McCullough, Robert Veatch, and me. In successive conferences we explored the history of how, in the eighteenth and nineteenth centuries, British and American physicians, philosophers and lawyers transformed medical manners and medical jurisprudence, into a new field that came to be called, "medical ethics."

R. Baker (✉)
Department of Philosophy, Union College, Schenectady, NY, USA
e-mail: bakerr@union.edu

L. M. Rasmussen, S. Holm (eds.), *50 Years of Philosophy and Medicine*,
Philosophy and Medicine 150, https://doi.org/10.1007/978-3-031-95175-6_7

Given the preponderance of historians participating in these conferences, we initially sought out scholarly presses specializing in the history of medicine. When these presses showed no interest in publishing our conference volumes, we turned to the founding editors of the Philosophy and Medicine series, Tris Engelhardt and Stuart Spicker. They welcomed the idea. So, curiously enough, a scholarly press dedicated to publishing works at the intersection of philosophy and medicine published bioethicists and historians of medicine's collaborative effort to develop a non-mythic history of how concepts and codes of medical ethics developed in the eighteenth and nineteenth century Anglophone medical cultures and lexicon.

Volume one, which came out in 1993, explored the emergence of "medical police" and codes of medical ethics as a response to the failure of eighteenth-century British and American medical etiquette to prevent physicians and surgeons' quarrels, "flytes" (a form of public verbal dueling), pamphlet wars, and duels. By January of 2024 this volume had been cited 44 times and was accessed online 966 times. Volume two focuses on subsequent nineteenth-century British and American developments in medical jurisprudence and medical ethics, and on the influence of Scottish moral sense theory on British-American medical morality. It has been cited 96 times and accessed 1563 times.

Once this precedent was set, I worked with fellow historically minded bioethicist, Laurence McCullough, to support other publications on the history of medical ethics. The next historical volume published in the Philosophy and Medicine series was McCullough's 1998 magisterial two-volume republication and study of the ethical works of the eighteenth-century Scottish enlightenment physician and philosopher, John Gregory, whose integration of moral sense theory into ideals of medical conduct influenced the development of medical morality in Britain and its colonies, including those in North America and Australia. As of January 2024, McCullough's edition of Gregory's writings (volume 57) had been cited 117 times and accessed online 1069 times; his companion book *John Gregory and the Invention of Professional Medical Ethics and the Profession of Medicine* (volume 56), has been cited 151 times, and accessed online 1099 times.

McCullough's republication of Gregory's writing set a precedent for reprinting historically important works in medical ethics. So, the next Philosophy and Medicine publication was William Stempsey's 2005 republication of nineteenth-century American physician Elisha Bartlett's 1844 book, *An Essay on the Philosophy of Medical Science* (volume 83). Reflecting the move to online publication, this volume was published as a hardback, a paperback, and an e-book. By January 2024, it had been accessed online 2832 times and had two citations. Similarly, Howard Brody, Zhara Meghani, and Kimberly Greenwald's 2009 publication of *Michael Ryan's Writings on Medical Ethics* was cited twice, but the online edition was accessed 6860 times. Dr. Ryan, a faculty member at the University of London's medical college, was notable for defending patients' rights to refuse to serve as research subjects. His defense of these rights was lampooned in *The Lancet*, as "Irish idiocy." As this comment indicates, Ryan also had to defend his right to respect as an Irish Catholic who presumed to teach ethics to English medical students in anti-Catholic nineteenth century Britain. As the first person to introduce the formal study of the writings of Gregory and Percival on "medical ethics" into a medical school's curriculum, Ryan was also the first person to have the official title "Professor of Medical Ethics."

In 2020 Lisa Rasmussen re-published the 1973 edition of Sir Kenneth Mellanby's *Human Guinea Pigs* (volume 134). In this edition, as in his best-selling 1945 edition, Mellanby proudly describes his use of World War II British conscientious objectors as human guinea pigs. In the 1973 edition Mellanby also defends the Nazi researchers condemned at the 1946 Nuremberg Medical Trial for their abusive exploitation of concentration camp internees as human guinea pigs. This third edition has two citations and was accessed online 5387 times.

Recognizing the endemic monolingualism of anglophone bioethicists, the Philosophy and Medicine series also publishes translations of important works published in other languages. Among these was the 2011 publication of, *Geschichte der Palliativmedizin: Medizinische Sterbebegleitung von 1500 bis heute*, by Michael Goldberg, MD, PhD, director of the *Institut für Geschichte der Medizin, Universität Würzburg* (Institute of the History of Medicine of Würzburg University). An updated and revised Philosophy and Medicine edition of Goldberg's history of palliative care was published in 2017 as, *A History of Palliative Care, 1500–1970: Concepts, Practices, and Ethical challenges* (volume 123). In this English translation Dr. Goldberg updates his account of the evolution and practice of palliative care, modern hospice movements, and medical aid in dying (MAID). The German edition has been cited 35 times, accessed 67 times; Philosophy and Medicine's English translation and update of the book has been cited 14 times and has been accessed over 12,000 times.

Perhaps the most challenging of the Philosophy and Medicine historical reprints is Melvin Wayne Cooper, MS (Bioethics), and MD's translation and reprint of a 1947 textbook by Rudolf Ramm, *SS-Standartenarzt* (SS physician), medical educator, and *Führer im Rasse-und Siedlungshauptam*t (Leader of the Central Department of Race and Settlements), *Ärztliche Rechts – und Standeskunde. Der Arzt als Gesundheitserzieh*, (volume 135). This Philosophy and Medicine translation was published in 2019 as *Medical Jurisprudence and the Rules of the Medical Profession*. While serving as a physician on a US military base in Germany, Dr. Cooper came across and read Ramm's textbook. He soon realized that it was the Nazi régime's official textbook of legal and ethical regulations for physicians, which was required reading for all medical students and healthcare professionals during the Nazi era. Given the textbook's role in acculturating German physicians in Nazi medical ethics and conditioning them to accept or participate in the Holocaust and the eugenic extermination of children with disabilities, Dr. Cooper believed it imperative to translate the book into English. He undertook on this task as his Masters of Bioethics project and, after graduating, spent decades refining the translation and footnoting it to make the text more accessible to twenty-first century readers. It has three citations was accessed 837 times.

The most recent publication in the history of medical ethics series is another magisterial study by Laurence McCullough; a 2022 book, *Thomas Percival's Medical Ethics and the Invention of Medical Professionalism* (volume 142). In this book McCullough reprints Percival's groundbreaking work, *Medical Ethics*, and several other ethically relevant writings, including Percival's book of morality tales for children. McCullough also explores why and how, in 1803, Percival introduced the concept of a code of professional medical ethics into the English language medical lexicon. He argues that, if one accepts Robert Baker's account of moral revolutions, Percival's book, *Medical Ethics*, and John Gregory's earlier writings were pivotal in a moral revolution in which medical ethics supplanted medical manners and etiquette as the morality of modern medicine.

In Greek myth and religion Zeus impregnated a goddess who gave birth in the usual manner to another daughter, Clio, the goddess of memory and history. In the *Nichomachean Ethics*, the Athenian philosopher, Aristotle, urged the transformation of memory into history through the systematic interrogations of information (data) by posing the following six questions: Who? What? Where? When? Why? and, How? St. Thomas Aquinas would later dub these questions the *Septem Circumstantiae.* Today such interrogations of memory in all its forms remain the backbone of historical scholarship, irrespective of whether these memories are preserved as emails, documents, images (e.g., in or on books, coin reliefs, newspapers, paintings, prints, sculptures, videos. etc.), letters, memorials, websites, and prior scholarly publications.

Bioethicists may still opt to embrace their inherited memories, their origin stories, uninterrogated by historians. If so their experiences and knowledge base will be limited to the present. Thus, to modify a well-known warning penned by a famous Hispanic American philosopher Jorge Agustín Nicolás Ruiz de Santayana y Borrás (better known in English as George Santayana), insofar as they ignorant of their history, "They are condemned to repeat it." For the past fifty years, history scholarship published in the Philosophy and Medicine series has preserved and interrogated memories of the past and will continue to do so to create the historical works that should enable bioethicists to understand their past, use this knowledge to better confront the present, and to more accurately anticipate the future.

Chapter 8
The Catholic Studies in Bioethics Subseries

Christopher Tollefsen

8.1 The Founders

To the best of my recollection, H. Tristram Engelhardt invited me to take over the editorship of the Catholic Studies in Bioethics (CSIB) subseries in 2001 or perhaps early 2002. The first volume under my editorship, *Pope John Paul II's Contribution to Catholic Bioethics* (which I edited) appeared in 2004; the last, and final in the series before its ending, was Jason Eberl's *Contemporary Controversies in Catholic Bioethics*, in 2017.[1] I'll return to my stewardship of the series shortly. But first, I'll discuss the origins of the series and the work of its early editors. Mapping the aspirations of the series founders will make possible an appraisal of continuities and discontinuities between the first ten years of the series' life and the remaining fifteen and a judgment of whether the series was overall successful by its own lights.

The Philosophy of Medicine series at the time was overseen by Engelhardt and S.F. Spicker. In a recent email to me, Fr. Kevin William Wildes, SJ, noted that Engelhardt saw an opportunity for a subseries on the Catholic moral tradition to publish work that did not fit neatly into the P & M series. In its initial run, Francesc Abel, SJ, and John Harvey were listed as subseries Editors, with Fr. Wildes identified as the Associate Editor. The first volume, which appeared in 1992, was titled *Birth, Suffering, and Death: Catholic Perspectives at the Edge of Life* and was listed as edited by all three, although with Fr. Wildes named as first editor. The volume

[1] See Appendix 1 for a complete list of the CSIB volumes. Although the subseries does not exist anymore as such, Eberl is joining the P&M series as an associate editor, and is currently at work on a volume on emerging issues in Catholic bioethics. Thus, I anticipate that the P&M series as a whole will continue to fulfill much of the mission of the subseries.

C. Tollefsen (✉)
Department of Philosophy, University of South Carolina, Columbia, SC, USA

L. M. Rasmussen, S. Holm (eds.), *50 Years of Philosophy and Medicine*, Philosophy and Medicine 150, https://doi.org/10.1007/978-3-031-95175-6_8

contains a Foreword by Edmund Pellegrino, a Preface by Abel and Harvey, and then a brief introductory essay by Wildes. Across these three brief pieces, I think we see four different justifications and explanations for the existence of a new subseries within the Philosophy and Medicine series.

Of least continuing relevance of these, but important to the actual history, was a pragmatic decision discussed by Abel and Harvey. In the 1980s, a body of scholars had formed the International Study Group on Bioethics to "promote dialogue among medical scientists on the one hand and Roman Catholic ethicists and moral theologians on the other" (Abel and Harvey 1992, xii). At the outset, "no record or proceedings" from the Group's meetings were published. But Abel and Harvey report that in consequence, "much valuable philosophical and theological reflection…was being lost" (Abel and Harvey 1992, xii). The CSIB subseries in the P&M series was thus conceived partly to create an outlet for publication of the fruits of these meetings. Fr. Wildes reports (again via email) that a Dutch foundation provided early funding for meetings of the Group that then led to content for early volumes, and the structure of the first volume reflects the nature of the Study Group, with an initial set of essays authored by medical professionals, and subsequent essays by philosophers and theologians.

When I inherited the editorship, however, Engelhardt made reference neither to the Study Group nor to potential sources of funding, and the series subsequently proceeded independently of any organized meetings by which to procure written content. It is very possible this was as much a feature of my relative juniority as of anything else; I only received tenure in 2002, and had not been trained in bioethics. I thus did not have the connections that might have made seeking funding a real possibility and did not give that much thought.

The three other justifications mentioned in the first volume were, however, to remain highly salient through the series' existence. First: in his "Forward," Pellegrino noted a shift in medical ethics from a time in which the preeminent, if not sole, voice of philosophical and theological reflection was Roman Catholic, to the (then) most recent two decades, in which the "center of gravity of ethical reflection shifted sharply", and the field had become dominated by secular thinkers. Pellegrino characterized the new approach to bioethics as "pluralistic, libertarian, and individualistic," "antipathetic to natural law arguments," and possessed of a relativistic and utilitarian ethos (Pellegrino 1992, ix). "Believers of whatever their persuasion are virtually disenfranchised in public policy debates" (Pellegrino 1992, x). Thus, CSIB was born in an attempt to offer "more visible, effective witness to the Catholic Perspective on Medical Morals" (Pellegrino 1992, x). Pellegrino's charter for this effort is worth quoting in full:

> To be effective that witness must be informed, intelligent, and scholarly. It must be in dialogue with the mainstream of thinkers in secular biomedical ethics. The Christian ethical points of view must be authentically, responsibly, and charitably presented. Such an effort must be international and trans-cultural, since medical progress presents a world-wide challenge to moral values (Pellegrino 1992, x).

So the CSIB series was, in Pellegrino's vision, an attempt to regain a "voice" for Catholic bioethics, a voice which, if adequately "informed, intelligent, and scholarly," might hope to be heard in the world in secular bioethics.

Fr Wildes articulates a second justification and aspiration for the series, deeply complementary to the first. In his introductory essay he speaks of the "experience of moral pluralism and the inability to speak in terms of a more fundamental, content-full universal narrative" (Wildes 1992a, 3). Wildes' essay, showing the influence of both Engelhardt (Wildes' advisor) and Alasdair MacIntyre, argues that "In the face of such cultural changes it becomes crucial for traditions, such as Catholicism, to reinterpret and rearticulate themselves so that they can understand themselves and speak to others" (Wildes 1992a, 3). In his subsequent essay in the volume on the good of human life, Wildes pursues this point in a critical engagement with the "New" Natural Law Theory:

> In a purely secular, pluralistic context, one finds numerous competing interpretations of human nature and basic human goods. One cannot choose among them without having already taken a particular moral stand. Finnis, Boyle, and Grisez need to acknowledge the extent to which their arguments are embedded within a particular moral tradition and its richness (Wildes 1992b, 147).

The CSIB subseries thus was understood by Wildes at least in part as an attempt to understand and articulate Roman Catholic bioethics self-consciously as a contentful moral tradition; Wildes saw this as a necessary condition for that tradition's being able, as Pellegrino hoped, to speak to other traditions.

Finally, Wildes identified a fourth aspiration or justification for the series, namely that the series bring the resources of the Catholic tradition to bear on emerging issues, especially those driven by technological change and exacerbated by the crisis of moral disagreement and pluralism. Accordingly, several chapters of the first volume addressed the question of providing nutrition and hydration to patients in a persistent vegetative state, an issue brought to prominence by the then still relatively recent cases of Karen Ann Quinlan and Nancy Cruzan.

How and to what extent did the series under my editorship succeed in realizing these goals? In the next three sections, I'll briefly discuss each relation to what I take to be some of paradigmatic books and essays that the CSIB subseries published between 2004 and 2017. I think there is a strong case to be made that the subseries both met the expectations of the early founders and provided and important scholarly and specifically Catholic voice in contemporary bioethics.

8.2 Reengaging with Secular Bioethics

Recall Pellegrino's concern that the voice of Catholic bioethics had been silenced in the secular world; he urged that reengagement was only possible through "informed, intelligent, and scholarly" interventions in which the Catholic view was authentically and charitably presented. To my mind, a central case of this effort is to be found in the volume edited by Stephen Napier in 2011, *Persons, Moral Worth, and Embryos: A Critical Analysis of Pro-Choice Arguments*.

As Napier makes clear, *Persons, Moral Worth, and Embryos* is an explicit attempt to engage dialectically with the philosophical consensus regarding embryonic and fetal human life. That consensus arose out of secular work in the philosophy of personal identity and in ethics that largely *preceded* philosophical explorations of the morality of abortion. In the realm of philosophy of mind, Napier identifies in particular the work of Sydney Shoemaker, who argued, using a particularly persuasive thought experiment involving brain swapping, for a psychological account of personal identity through time (an account indebted to John Locke and Locke's own ingenious thought experiments). It is a short step from such an account, for which psychological connectedness is a necessary condition of the identity of persons through time, to the view that an entity with no psychological states is not the kind of thing with which a person *can* be trans-temporally identical. Accordingly, embryos and fetuses, which have no or few psychological states, are not persons.

In ethics and the philosophy of value, Napier again notes philosophical currents preceding the abortion debate that nevertheless influenced it. The dialectic described in the paragraphs above concern what it means, metaphysically, to be a person through time. But one could detach concerns about moral status from questions about the essential nature of beings such as the readers and author of this essay, and use the word "person" less as a designator of a being's essential *nature* and more as a marker for whether a being's life matters in the ways relevant to the abortion controversy. If a being possesses the kind of moral status according to which it would be wrong to kill that being at will, or for the sake of benefits that would accrue only to another, then such a being would be designated a person. But any being not possessing such a moral status, including, potentially, some human beings, would fail to be a person in this moral sense.

Such a distinction could emerge in view of axiological claims about the link between "intrinsic value and consciousness," and Napier demonstrates in his introduction that once again the philosophical path was paved prior to the beginnings of serious debate about abortion, in work going back to G.E. Moore, and cited approvingly later in the century by Brand Blandshard: "Moore's final conclusion was, then, that a universe without consciousness would be a universe without value. With this I think we must agree" (Blanshard 1961, p. 273).

That there is a link between this claim about the value of consciousness and claims to the non-valuable standing of embryos and fetuses seems plausible. It is not long into the abortion debate that philosophers such as Mary Ann Warren and Michael Tooley are found denying that moral status could belong to a being not yet possessed of sentience or sapience, a view refined and defended with great skill and subtlety by later philosophers such as Jeff McMahan, David DeGrazia, and David Boonin. A particularly prominent version of this view holds that because fetuses do not and cannot *take* an interest in remaining alive, that therefore their being killed is not a harm to them (discussed at some length in Tollefsen 2011).

The various essays in Napier's book engage head-on with this array of secular, mainstream, philosophical arguments, all of which can reasonably be described as forming the professional philosophic "consensus" on the question of abortion. Napier's authors, such as Alexander Pruss, Jason Eberl, and Francis Beckwith, argue against the metaphysical claim concerning personhood by defending in one form or another the view now known as "animalism", which holds that you, the reader of this essay, and I, the author, are essentially animal organisms, namely, human beings. Thus, as Pruss argues, it is true of me, and for you, that each of us was "once a fetus" (Pruss 2011).

Likewise, Pruss and Napier's authors, including myself, argue that fetuses are possessed of full moral status, that their lives are of intrinsic value, and that killing fetuses is wrong in the same circumstances generally that killing other human beings is. Each essay in the section of Napier's volume titled "Philosophical Considerations" engages at length with the best and most rigorous arguments that secular metaphysics and moral philosophy has to offer (with David Hershenov even writing about the implications of four-dimensionalism about time in his essay).

I would note another important feature of the Napier volume as regards this issue of engagement with secular bioethics. If you and I are human beings, and all human beings possess a right not to be killed at will, then it is essential to the debate about both abortion and embryo destructive research that we possess a sound account of when human beings begin. Many of the authors of Napier's volume have, in various places, addressed this question, understanding it as fundamentally a question of biological fact, not one of speculative metaphysics. Maureen Condic's contribution to the volume, "A Biological Definition of the Human Embryo," looks at this question from the standpoint of developmental biology, proposing a definition that takes account of both function and composition, and demonstrates, convincingly to my mind, that most human embryos begin their lives with "the fusion of sperm and egg plasma membranes" (Condic 2011, 222). Her essay is essential reading for anyone who wants to engage with this biological question in a scientifically informed manner.

The view that you and I are essentially human beings; that human beings by their nature are possessed of a rational nature; and that all beings possessed of a rational nature possess a fundamental right to life, is often referred to as the "Substantial Identity View," so called because moral status is said to depend on one's identity as a being of a certain kind of (rational) substance (in this case, human being). Some of the most prominent defenders of that position were contributors to Napier's and other volumes of the series, including Francis Beckwith (to the Napier volume); Patrick Lee and Joseph Boyle (to multiple volumes – together they are the most prolific authors in the subseries); and Robert P. George (to the *festschrift* for Joseph Boyle, *Bioethics with Liberty and Justice: Themes in the Work of Joseph M. Boyle*). The Substantial Identity View is one of the two major competitors to the consensus view on which human beings lack intrinsic value and rights prior to the achievement of some state of consciousness.

The other competitor view is that of Donald Marquis, dubbed by him the "Future of Value View" (Marquis 1989). On Marquis's account, abortion is wrong because it deprives a fetus of a future of value, a future that, it could reasonably be expected, would be full of many worthwhile experiences. Intuitively, such a view differs from the substantial identity view less in its claims about abortion than, e.g., in its claims about euthanasia and physician assisted suicide, particularly in cases in which the subject of the death would soon die anyway.

The Boyle *festschrift* is notable for an extended discussion between Marquis, criticizing the view of Boyle, Beckwith, Lee, and George, and Lee and Boyle themselves. As Boyle notes, the exchange marks an important contribution to the debate, with Marquis leveling a number of criticisms of the Substantial Identity View, and Lee providing significant refinements of the theory in response (Marquis 2012; Lee 2012). For example: a claim of the Substantial Identity View is that certain rights, which are possessed universally and invariantly by all mature human beings, such as the right not to be enslaved, or killed at will, must be based on properties that are themselves universal and invariant across all the beings who possess those rights. Thus, proponents hold, the right should be based not on properties such as the developed ability to engage in this or that feature of cognition or volition, since that ability comes in degrees and sometimes not at all, but rather on the possession of a rational nature, which does not come in degrees and is of course possessed by every being with that kind of nature.

Marquis interprets the Substantial Identity View as saying that there are two kinds of capacities, basic natural capacities, and developed capacities. Since the latter, on his understanding of the argument, exist on a continuum, they are inappropriate bases for a right to life. But, objects Marquis, such capacities do not exist on a continuum throughout an individual's life, since they do not exist early in a human being's life at all. Moreover, capacities of the first sort (natural capacities) do not exist equally in all human individuals, even from the beginning, since some humans are "naturally dim-witted and some are naturally smart." So the Substantial Identity View's effort to find a strong contrast between a property that exists everywhere on a continuum and a single universal and equally held property fails.

Lee's clarifications are subtle and complex, and not easily summarized here; but the two crucial points are these. First, there are not in fact two different capacities, a natural one, and a developed one. Rather, the developed capacity just is the natural capacity *at some particular stage of development and expression.* Second, that a being has a natural capacity for rational thought *is* a capacity held equally and essentially by all beings that have it, even if other accidental properties prevent (or foster) a fuller expression of that capacity. Thus, as Lee writes,

> Having basic rights – moral immunity from being killed or enslaved, the right to be treated as others would have themselves be treated – follows upon being an individual with a rational nature, not on the possession of a degree of some property (such as the immediately exercisable capacity for reasoning), nor on factors in one's constitution that will aid or impede the more complete development of one's rational nature (Lee 2012, 30).

It is fair to say of Marquis's Future of Value View that it is the most prominent secular "pro-life" approach to abortion, converging with a "Catholic" view in its conclusion, but departing in its starting point. The dialogue between Marquis, on the one hand, and a large number of contributors to the CSIB subseries marks, in my view, a significant achievement in relation to Pellegrino's desire that the series serve to restore Catholic moral thought to the domain of secular moral discussion.

8.3 Interpreting and Articulating the Tradition

Fr Kevin William Wildes identified a second motivation for the series and a benchmark by which entries in the series might be assessed, namely that, in cultural conditions of pluralism and disagreement, "it becomes crucial for traditions, such as Catholicism, to reinterpret and rearticulate themselves so that they can understand themselves and speak to others" (Wildes 1992a, 3).

It is perhaps worth saying a bit about the roots this idea has in the thought of Alasdair MacIntyre, whom Wildes cites approvingly. In *After Virtue*, MacIntyre described a crisis in what he later came to call, with Bernard Williams, "the morality system." For centuries, according to MacIntyre, philosophers had attempted to justify "morality" in a way that was in principle available for agreement and acquiescence by anyone, anywhere. Such justifications would presuppose no cultural, historical, or religious tradition, and indeed, philosophy in service to the "Enlightenment Project" of providing such a form of justification has been and remains deeply suspicious of tradition (MacIntyre 1984).

Yet, MacIntyre argued, the concepts and language of morality themselves grew out of particular cultural, historical, and ultimately religious contexts and traditions, especially those of ancient Greece, Israel, and eventually Western Christianity. Shorn of that complicated and multi-faceted context, justification becomes impossible, and moral philosophy practically becomes, on MacIntyre's telling, bankrupt. Moral language itself is available only as a means of furthering the expression of one's emotions.

Macintyre's *Whose Justice, Which Rationality*? probed deeper into what it means for a morality's understanding of justice and practical rationality to be embedded and intelligible within a tradition (MacIntyre 1988). Sympathetic entry into, if not first-person life within, a moral tradition is a necessary condition for being able to understand its conceptual apparatus and language and to begin both to articulate that tradition, and to identify and overcome internal challenges to it, such as disagreement between inhabitants of the tradition.

MacIntyre went still further in *Whose Justice*. Talk of tradition-bound rationalities and justices seems dangerously close to relativism, a danger compounded by MacIntyre's tendency to speak of "rival and incommensurable" traditions. Indeed, Bernard Williams, who is similar to MacIntyre in various ways, was himself deeply skeptical of the claim that one tradition could be vindicated in relation to another sufficiently alien moral tradition. One might tell a historical story about how, say, a Roman world in which political authority was insensitive to the ideal of democratic voice, human equality, and political representation had disappeared, to be replaced by a Western world of liberal democracy and human dignity, but that story would not be one of vindication (Williams 2006).

In *Whose Justice*, MacIntyre forwarded an account both of how internal tensions and errors in a tradition of moral enquiry might be overcome, such that a tradition might be said to make intellectual progress, and also of how two "rival and incommensurable" moral traditions might come into *rational* conflict, so that one tradition might be vindicated in relation to another. The first kind of progress is a necessary condition for the second and requires:

- That later stages of the enquiry presuppose the findings of the earlier stages while being able to explain instances of irresolvable disagreement at earlier stages (MacIntyre 1988, 79–80);
- That later stages provide a "successively more adequate account of the good of the enquiry" and an increasingly adequate idea of what it would be mean to complete the enquiry is developed (MacIntyre 1988, 80);
- That the correction of false views comes with an explanation of why such false views might be expected if the overall standpoint was correct (MacIntyre 1988, 118);
- And that there be genuine confrontation between rival views within the tradition "so that we may arrive at a conclusion as to which of these best survives the strongest objections which can be advanced on the basis of the others" (MacIntyre 1988, 118).

All this both as prolegomenon to entering into genuine conflict with rival views, and as essential to a tradition's being able "to reinterpret and rearticulate "itself.

To a MacIntyrean, it might seem that my description of the series' efforts to pit the Catholic moral tradition against the secular "philosophical consensus" on a matter such as abortion put the engagement cart before the interpretive horse. But in fact, the work of engaging with secular culture went hand in hand, in the subseries' development, with the work of understanding, interpreting, and articulating the Catholic tradition of moral enquiry from within, and of engaging at the same time in the work of sustaining "genuine confrontation" between rival views within that tradition. Nowhere is this clearer that in the recurrence, constantly within the subseries, of work on the question of nutrition and hydration.

Several chapters of the inaugural volume of the subseries had already addressed the question of providing nutrition and hydration to patients in a persistent vegetative state, an issue brought to initial prominence by the cases of Karen Ann Quinlan and Nancy Cruzan, and later by the case of Theresa Schiavo, and with a rich history of discussion within Roman Catholicism. The consensus view taken in the first volume, *Birth, Suffering, and Death: Catholic Perspectives at the Edges of Life,* was that for patients in a persistent vegetative state, provision of nutrition and hydration by artificial means, such as a PEG tube, typically constituted "extraordinary" means – means that could, reasonably, be rejected and which are not obligatory to provide or accept. The essays of the volume are a window into the state of the Catholic debate in the 1990s: almost each essay to address the question of tube feeding of PVS patients takes aim at either Germain Grisez or those with whom he worked, as among the few representatives of the view that tube feeding was in most circumstances obligatory for patients in a persistent vegetative state. In that volume, Porter Storey, Benedict Ashley, O.P., Paul Schotsman, Kevin Wildes, S.J., Thomas Bole, and John Paris, S.J. all argued that ANH should be considered an extraordinary, non-obligatory form of care. No author in the volume took the contrary position (Storey, 1992; Ashley 1992; Wildes 1992b; Bole 1992; Paris 1992).

The dominance of that position was challenged twelve years later in 2004 with Pope John Paul II's address, "Care for Patients in the Permanent Vegetative State." In that allocution, the Pope announced that providing artificial nutrition and hydration to patients in a PVS should be considered "ordinary care" and thus in principle obligatory:

> I should like to underline how the administration of food and water, even when provided by artificial means, always represents a natural means of preserving life, not a medical act. Its use, furthermore, should be considered, in principle, ordinary and proportionate, and as such morally obligatory, insofar as and until it is seen to have attained its proper finality, which in the present case consists in providing nourishment to the patient and alleviation of his suffering (John Paul II 2004, no. 4).

The Pope went on to warn that withdrawal of ANH from such patients "ends up becoming, if done knowingly and willingly, true and proper euthanasia by omission" (John Paul II 2004, no. 4). According to one commentator, the document "sent shock waves through the Catholic health care system," prompting a widespread rethinking of the ethics of ANH (Hamel 2007).

Happily, the subseries was perfectly poised to contribute this debate. That same year, I had edited *John Paul II's Contribution to Catholic Bioethics*. The volume contained probing essays on the Pope's philosophical and theological treatments of the good of human life, the importance of the human body and of human relationality and sexuality, and deep investigations into John Paul's personalism. These were written by top Catholic bioethicists, including Luke Gormally, Patrick Lee, and Andrew Lustig, among others, who all made clear just how central a figure in Catholic bioethics the Pope had become. The volume also included prominent non-Catholic voices such as Michael Murray, Mark Cherry, and Joel Shuman, reflecting my desire that the series make possible engagement between Catholics and other Christians both on matters of agreement and disagreement.

Following the publication of Christopher Kaczor's monograph, *The Edge of Life* in 2005, the third volume under my series editorship addressed the papal allocution head on. *Artificial Nutrition and Hydration: The New Catholic Debate* contains contributions from many of the leading defenders of the Pope's allocution, as well as an exchange between perhaps the most prominent critic of the Pope's allocution, Fr. Kevin O'Rourke, and defenders Patrick Lee and Mark Latkovic.

It is worth spending some time on the essays from this volume, for it contains, in my opinion, some of the best Catholic writing on that topic, much or all of which tracks the MacIntyrean aspiration to interpret, understand and articulate the Catholic tradition, while overcoming internal disagreement and furthering the goal of progress in moral enquiry.

Consider, for example, then Bishop (now Archbishop of Sydney) Anthony Fisher's "Why Do Unresponsive Patients Still Matter?" (Fisher 2008). Fisher's essay exemplifies the principle, articulated by John Paul II in his encyclical *Fides et Ratio,* that the Catholic tradition, including its moral tradition, breathes through "two lungs", faith and reason. Thus, genuine Catholic teaching on the matter of artificial provision of nutrition and hydration should be expected to find support both in positive natural law argument and dialectical exchange with other moral approaches, and in the revelation of Scripture.

Bishop Fisher thus proceeds first to identify the philosophical anthropology that underlies the claim that unresponsive patients still "matter" – *pace* the work of secular thinkers such as Ronald Dworkin. Rather than see human beings as of value merely insofar as they are loci for autonomous choice in pursuit of personal preference, so that severely debilitated human beings would no longer count as persons, the Catholic approach sees the moral life as guided by objective moral norms, and the human being as possessed of an intrinsic value and dignity. Bishop Fisher's discussion of the philosophical dialectic on this topic repays study.

It is, however, on the theological side that Bishop Fisher's essay is most noteworthy. Fisher notes that all religions are concerned in some way with eating and feeding. But Christianity goes much further:

> In fact the turning points of Jesus' life are always marked by eating and drinking. His first great sign is turning water into wine; his first preaching to a gentile began with a request for a drink and ended with a promise of endless living water; his most recorded miracle is the multiplication of loaves and fishes; his last wonder before his ascension is the huge haul of fish (Mt 14:13ff par; Jn 2:1ff; Chaps. 4 and 21). All these miracles were of end-time proportions, divine in their extravagance, a foretaste of the longed-for messianic banquet (Isa 25:6–8; 1 Sam 2:5; Lk 1:53). As his ministry
>
> came to its climax, he took his closest friends aside for a last meal, investing the Passover Seder with new significance: his own Pasch memorialized and perpetuated in the Eucharist (Mt 26:20ff par; cf. Jn Chaps. 6 and 13). Before returning to the Father he dined again with disoriented disciples in Emmaus, with confused apostles at the Sunday gathering and with his nearest and dearest at the lakeside breakfast in Galilee (Lk 24:13ff; Mk 16:14; Jn Chap. 21) (Fisher 2008, 23).

From these and other Scriptural observations, Fisher begins to provide a theology of eating and of feeding, and the relation of these to questions of power, service, dependence, community, in and out-groups, and ultimately of salvation. It is an exemplary instance of the working out in the Catholic moral tradition of the implications of an elemental but often overlooked intersection between our quotidian life and the life of Jesus in the Gospels, and is one of the essays I am most proud to have published in my time as series editor.

The virtues of *Artificial Nutrition and Hydration: The New Catholic Debate* are not exhausted by Bishop Fisher's essay, however. Beyond a number of philosophically sophisticated essays by thinkers such as Joseph Boyle, J.L.A. Garcia, and Peter Cataldo, and a helpful tour of the relevant legal questions by Jacqueline Laing, the volume also includes the aforementioned exchange between Fr. O'Rourke and Patrick Lee and Mark Latkovic. Considerations of space will not allow me to do justice to the dialectic, but the four essays in this part of the volume together constitute precisely that genuine confrontation between rival views within a tradition that MacIntyre believes enable us to "arrive at a conclusion as to which of these best survives the strongest objections which can be advanced on the basis of the other." I will leave it to readers to judge which position on this matter does best survive the objections of the other, but I trust they will agree with the following: by the second,

MacIntyrean, measure of success proposed by Fr Wildes, the subseries should be judged a success.

8.4 Addressing New Issues

In his introduction to the first volume of the subseries, Fr Wildes spoke of the need for Catholic bioethics to be "responsive to new needs and challenges," and of the dilemmas raised by modern medical practice. This requires an orientation backwards, towards the tradition from which Catholic bioethicists draw their resources, and forwards, to creative engagement with emerging issues. This Janus-faced orientation of Catholic bioethics is evident enough in the topic discussed at such length in the previous section, artificial nutrition and hydration. Catholic attention to the ethics of eating and feeding is hardly new; as Fr. Daniel Cronin (subsequently the Archbishop of Hartford) discussed in his 1958 dissertation, republished as *Ordinary and Extraordinary Means of Conserving* Life, discussion of circumstances under which it is permissible to refuse life-sustaining nourishment goes back at least to Francisco de Vitoria, who wrote in his *Relectiones Theologicae*:

> If a sick man can take food or nourishment with a certain hope of life, he is required to take food as he would be required to give it to one who is sick. However, if the depression of spirits is so severe and there is present grave consternation in the appetitive power so that only with the greatest effort and as though through torture can the sick man take food, this is to be reckoned as an impossibility and therefore, he is excused, at least from mortal sin (quoted on 49–50 of Cronin 2011).

But Vitoria was, obviously, not familiar with the opportunities and challenges presented by modern medicine with its capacity to sustain a non-responsive patient for perhaps years through the artificial administration of nutrition and hydration. The tradition required development.

Nor, as we have also seen, was that development without disagreement. Core principles such as the sanctity of human life and the ordinary-extraordinary means distinction can be held by all, yet the understandings and applications of such principles can differ even among Catholic thinkers of sound faith and good will. Thus we again return to MacIntyre's dictum that progress in a tradition requires the articulation and prosecution of even vigorous disagreements.

And so, in pursuit of the third desideratum of the Catholic Studies in Bioethics subseries, that the Catholic tradition be brought to bear on new and emerging issues, it is unsurprising that we find once again an attempt as well to articulate and interpret the tradition in its bearing on what, even within the Catholic tradition, are at present deeply contested questions. To give two examples:

First, 2008 saw, in addition to the volume on nutrition and hydration, a volume edited by Sarah-Vaughan Brakman and Darlene Fozard Weaver, *The Ethics of Embryo Adoption and the Catholic Tradition*, which addressed an issue scarcely conceivable to Catholics prior to the advent in the 1960s and 70s of radically new technologies for assisted reproduction, especially *in vitro* fertilization. In consequence of the way in which IVF is conducted, which typically involves numerous "spare" embryos left unimplanted and stored in cryopreservation, a question had arisen for Catholic bioethics about the appropriate response to these embryonic human beings.

For, on the one hand, as we have seen in our discussion of Bishop Fisher and elsewhere, the Catholic moral tradition is unequivocal in holding that there is a dignity and sanctity to every individual human being, and that positive obligations are owed for the care and preservation of human life (e.g., by feeding). On the other hand, less discussed in this essay, but well known, the Catholic moral tradition's understanding of the sanctity of *marriage* has consequences for how children should come into existence. As the Congregation for the Doctrine of the Faith put it, "[t]he bond existing between husband and wife accords the spouses, in an objective and inalienable manner, the exclusive right to become father and mother solely through each other" (CDF 1987, II.A.2).

This injunction has been taken as an obstacle to the proposal made by some, in defense of the lives of cryopreserved and abandoned human embryos, that they be saved from their "absurd" fate by being rescued or adopted: transferred into the womb of a willing woman and perhaps adopted by the gestating mother along with her husband. This is clearly oriented towards the good of an unborn human being, and seems in accord with the Catholic understanding of the sanctity even of embryonic human life. But does such a proposal violate the norm that spouses become "father and mother solely through each other," given the intervention of a medical technician and the lack of a biological relationship between the parents and the implanted embryo?

Though perhaps less vigorous now, the early 2000s were dominated, in the world of Catholic bioethics, by discussion of this question, which raises questions of act analysis, the nature of adoptive parenthood, and pro-life witness. Brakman and Weaver accordingly brought forth a volume in which both sides saw equal representation in an effort to get the best available arguments for and against "embryo adoption" in conversation with one another. They also brought into the conversation Protestant thinkers, such as Eric Gregory (Protestants had been generally supportive of embryo adoption, while theorizing about it somewhat less than Catholics) and practitioners of embryo adoption, both on the medical side, and on the parental side. Thus their volume uniquely addressed both theoretical and experiential aspects of the question, setting a high mark of scholarly excellence in the treatment of a relatively novel issue. This volume remains an invaluable resources for those working on this issue, and I have consulted it myself in recent work on this issue.

Which leads me to the final volume of the series, *Contemporary Controversies in Catholic Bioethics*, edited by Jason Eberl. As the title indicates, this volume was explicitly conceived as an effort to bring together Catholic bioethicists who, while agreeing at some level of principle, had not yet achieved agreement on emerging and essential issues in Catholic medicine. Eberl's volume contains forty essays over seven parts, with each part organized around a disputed issue, and framed in each case with a helpful introductory section by Eberl outlining "the history of how the issues treated therein emerged and have been addressed by both secular authorities and the Catholic magisterium" (Eberl 2017, 4). The volume is "intended to provide an up-to-date resource for both Catholic and non-Catholic scholars of the various debated issues treated herein, each author marshalling the latest scientific information, philosophical and theological arguments, and Catholic magisterial teaching to make the case for their respective conclusions" (Eberl 2017, 4).

And thus we return full circle to the three aspirations and benchmarks for judgment of the series: Catholic engagement with the secular world of bioethics, Catholic articulation and interpretation of the tradition, including vigorous intra-traditional argument, and Catholic grappling with new and emerging issues. To my mind, Eberl's volume encapsulates everything that the subseries founders aspired for the series to be and that I strove to realize over the fifteen years and ten volumes that I was its editor. Abel, Harvey, Wildes, and Engelhardt put into motion an intellectual and moral venture that bore significant fruit; the many authors and editors of the subseries and of the Philosophy and Medicine series more generally are due considerable gratitude for their contributions to realizing the goals of the series founders. Working with all of them to make that happen was a great privilege.

Appendix 1 Volumes Published in the Catholic Studies in Bioethics Subseries

Wildes, K.W., SJ, Abel, F., SJ, and Harvey, J.C., Eds. 1992. *Birth, Suffering, and Death: Catholic Perspectives at the Edge of Life.*

Wildes, K. W., SJ, Ed. 1995. *Critical Choices and Critical Care: Catholic Perspectives on Allocating Resources in Intensive Care Medicine.*

Wildes, K.W., SJ, Ed. 1997. *Infertility: A Crossroad of Faith, Medicine, and Technology*

Tollefsen, C., Ed. 2004. *John Paul II's Contribution to Catholic Bioethics*

Kaczor, C. 2005. *The Edge of Life: Human Dignity and Contemporary Bioethics*

Tollefsen, C. Ed. 2008. *Artificial Nutrition and Hydration: the New Catholic Debate*

Brakman, S.V. and Weaver, D.F., Eds. 2008. *The Ethics of Embryo Adoption and the Catholic Tradition*

Napier, S., Ed. 2011. *Persons, Moral Worth, and Embryos: A Critical Analysis of Pro-Choice Arguments*

Mazur, G., O.P. 2011. *Informed Consent, Proxy Consent, and Catholic Bioethics: For the Good of the Subject*

Tollefsen, C., Ed. 2012. *Bioethics with Liberty and Justice: Themes in the Work of Joseph M. Boyle*

Taboada, P., Ed. *Sedation at the End-of-life: An Interdisciplinary Approach*

Sobiech, F. 2016. *Ethos, Bioethics, and Sexual Ethics in Work and Reception of the Anatomist Niels Stensen (1638–1686)*

Eberl, J., Ed. 2017. *Contemporary Controversies in Catholic Bioethics*

References

Ashley, B. M. 1992. Dominion or Stewardship? Theological Reflections. In *Birth, Suffering, and Death: Catholic Perspectives at the Edge of Life*, ed. S. J. Kevin William Wildes, S. J. Francesc Abel, and J. C. Harvey, 85–106. Dordrecht, The Netherlands: Kluwer.

Blanshard, B. 1961. *Reason and Goodness*. London: George Allen and Unwin.

Bole, T. J. 1992. Why Almost Any Cost to Others to Preserve the Life of the Irreversibly Comatose Constitutes an Extraordinary Burden. In *Birth, Suffering, and Death: Catholic Perspectives at the Edge of Life*, ed. S. J. Kevin William Wildes, S. J. Francesc Abel, and J. C. Harvey, 171–187. Dordrecht, The Netherlands: Kluwer.

Condic, M. 2011. A Biological Definition of the Human Embryo. In *Persons, Moral Worth, and Embryos: A Critical Analysis of Pro-Choice Arguments*, ed. S. Napier, 211–235. Dordrecht, The Netherlands: Springer.

Congregation for the Doctrine of the Faith (CDF). 1987. *Donum Vitae* (February 22).

Cronin, D. A. 2011. *Ordinary and Extraordinary Means of Conserving Life*. Philadelphia, PA: The National Catholic Bioethics Center.

Eberl, J. 2017. Introduction. In *Contemporary Controversies in Catholic Bioethics*, ed. J. Eberl, 1–5. Dordrecht, The Netherlands: Springer.

Fisher, B. A. 2008. Why Do Unresponsive Patients Still Matter? In *Artificial Nutrition and Hydration: The New Catholic Debate*, ed. C. Tollefsen, 3–37. Dordrecht, The Netherlands: Springer.

Abel, F. S. J., and J. C. Harvey. 1992. Preface. In *Birth, Suffering, and Death: Catholic Perspectives at the Edge of Life*, ed. S. J. Kevin William Wildes, S. J. Francesc Abel, and J. C. Harvey, xi–xv. Dordrecht, The Netherlands: Kluwer.

Hamel, R. 2007. The Catholic Health Association's Response to the Papal Allocution on Artificial Nutrition and Hydration. *AMA Journal of Ethics* 9:388–392.

John Paris, S. J. 1992. The Catholic Tradition on the Use of Nutrition and Fluids. In *Birth, Suffering, and Death: Catholic Perspectives at the Edge of Life*, ed. S. J. Kevin William Wildes, S. J. Francesc Abel, and J. C. Harvey, 189–208. Dordrecht, The Netherlands: Kluwer.

John Paul, I. I. 2004. Care for Patients in the Permanent Vegetative State. *Origins 33*:738–740.

Kevin William Wildes, S. J. 1992a. Finitude, Religion, and Medicine: The Search for Meaning in the Post-Modern World. In *Birth, Suffering, and Death: Catholic Perspectives at the Edge of Life*, ed. S. J. Kevin William Wildes, S. J. Francesc Abel, and J. C. Harvey, 1–7. Dordrecht, The Netherlands: Kluwer.

Kevin William Wildes, S. J. 1992b. Life as a Good and Our Obligations to Persistently Vegetative Patients. In *Birth, Suffering, and Death: Catholic Perspectives at the Edge of Life*, ed. S. J. Kevin William Wildes, S. J. Francesc Abel, and J. C. Harvey, 145–154. Dordrecht, The Netherlands: Kluwer.

Lee, P. 2012. Substnatial Identity, Rational Nature, and the Right to Life. In *Bioethics with Liberty and Justice: Themes in the Work of Joseph M. Boyle*, ed. C. Tollefsen, 23–40. Doredrecht, The Netherlands: Springer.

MacIntyre, A. 1984. *After Virtue: A Study in Moral Theory*. 2nd ed. Notre Dame, IN: University of Notre Dame Press.

MacIntyre, A. 1988. *Whose Justice, Which Rationality?* Notre Dame, IN: University of Notre Dame Press.

Marquis, D. 1989. Why Abortion is Immoral. *The Journal of Philosophy* 86:138–202.

Marquis, D. 2012. Why Abortion is Seriously Wrong: Two Views. In *Bioethics with Liberty and Justice: Themes in the Work of Joseph M. Boyle*, ed. C. Tollefsen, 3–22. Dordrecht, The Netherlands: Springer.

Pellegrino, E. D. 1992. Foreward. In *Birth, Suffering, and Death: Catholic Perspectives at the Edge of Life*, ed. S. J. Kevin William Wildes, S. J. Francesc Abel, and J. C. Harvey, ix–x. Dordrecht, The Netherlands: Kluwer.

Pruss, A. 2011. I Was Once a Fetus: That Is Why Abortion Is Wrong. In *Persons, Moral Worth, and Embryos: A Critical Analysis of Pro-Choice Arguments*, ed. S. Napier, 19–42. Dordrecht, The Netherlands: Springer.

Storey, P. 1992. Artificial Feeding and Hydration in Advanced Illness. In *Birth, Suffering, and Death: Catholic Perspectives at the Edge of Life*, ed. S. J. Kevin William Wildes, S. J. Francesc Abel, and J. C. Harvey, 67–75. Dordrecht, The Netherlands: Kluwer.

Tollefsen, C. 2011. Fetal Persons, Fetal Interests, and Fetal Goods. In *Persons, Moral Worth, and Embryos: A Critical Analysis of Pro-Choice Arguments*, ed. S. Napier, 163–184. Dordrecht, The Netherlands: Springer.

Williams, B. 2006. *Philosophy as a Humanistic Discipline*. In *Philosophy as a Humanistic Discipline*, ed. A. W. Moore, 180–199. Princeton, NJ: Princeton University.

Chapter 9
The Place of the Family in East Asian Bioethics

Dawei Pan and Ruiping Fan

9.1 Introduction

During the past several decades, the world has witnessed the increased awareness of the significance of philosophical investigations into the domains of life science and healthcare, as illustrated by the "Philosophy and Medicine" (P&M) series by Springer. Among the almost 150 volumes in the series, there has been a special outpouring of interest regarding East Asian contributions to bioethics. Initiated in 1999, the P&M Asian subseries primarily aimed to provide readers a way to understand moral and cultural issues involved in healthcare, particularly in East Asian contexts. Over time, it has revealed an intriguing perspective on the development of a culturally sensitive approach to bioethics known as the family-based approach. This approach becomes particularly relevant in an era of growing cross-cultural exchanges, communication, and global political tensions, like the one we are currently experiencing.

Although those engaged in this approach are primarily philosophers and ethicists, they face a special and delicate challenge that is somewhat similar to that of an anthropologist, as depicted by Clifford Geertz. To meet this challenge, presumably, as Geertz (1988) puts it, simultaneously requires both the conviction of a

D. Pan (✉)
Department of Philosophy and Philosophy of Medicine Laboratory, Sun Yat-sen University, Guangzhou, China
e-mail: pandw@mail.sysu.edu.cn

R. Fan
Department of Public and International Affairs, City University of Hong Kong, Kowloon Tong, Hong Kong, China
e-mail: safan@cityu.edu.hk

L. M. Rasmussen, S. Holm (eds.), *50 Years of Philosophy and Medicine*, Philosophy and Medicine 150, https://doi.org/10.1007/978-3-031-95175-6_9

pilgrim and the dispassionate assessment of a cartographer.[1] Two closely interwoven questions are raised throughout the P&M Asian subseries: (1) How do the authors of the volumes establish their own identities as Asian or Asian-based bioethicists? (2) What research are they expected to perform? The first question is a matter of constructing a scholarly identity, notably one that is connected to the international community of bioethics while at the same time that has its own "signature," or, rather, perhaps its own unique "Asian" or "Confucian" identity.[2] Such an identity is critical for the researchers not only because contentious moral issues are nearly always involved in a variety of specific contexts and appeal to historic precedent and cultural heritage rather than to abstract principles. More importantly, like anthropologists, ethicists and philosophers concerning themselves with real issues must stay in the real world and be there for people instead of detaching themselves from it to get a better understanding of what humanities scholars can do in and for it. The second pertains to developing a way that aligns with this identity in the academic world. The first brings charges of certitude, of finding one's own voice, making a trenchant stand, and arguing about normative matters or even cultural or spiritual commitments. The second question calls for objectivity to tell the truth about the ongoing reality in their areas' healthcare and bioethical issues, of revealing true evidence for the existence of a distinctively East Asian Confucian ethos.

The creative tension between Asian or Asian-based bioethicists as pilgrims and as cartographers runs throughout all of the nearly dozen volumes of the Asian Subseries under the P&M series. This approach begins with an elucidation of concerns about moral differences, or even conflicts between cultures or religions, followed by inquiries and evaluations to address these concerns in empirically sound and increasingly precise ways. The early exploration of the approach can be dated back to 61st P&M volume titled *Confucian Bioethics* (1999) edited by Ruiping Fan

[1] Geertz argues that conducting anthropological research necessitates embodying the conviction of a pilgrim and the dispassionate assessment of a cartographer. The metaphor of a pilgrim refers to the researcher's immersion in the culture they study, adopting a genuine curiosity and openness to understanding it from within. This perspective allows the researcher to grasp the meanings and values that shape the cultural practices and beliefs of the community being studied. On the other hand, the metaphor of a cartographer highlights the need for a certain level of detachment and objectivity. Like a mapmaker, the researcher must carefully observe, document, and analyze the cultural phenomena without imposing personal biases or judgments. The difference lies in the balancing act between immersion and detachment. Geertz suggests that anthropologists should immerse themselves in the culture they study to gain a deep understanding, but they should also maintain a critical distance to avoid becoming overly subjective or romanticizing the culture. This approach allows for a nuanced and comprehensive analysis of the cultural context. See Geertz (1988, p. 10). Although the East Asian scholars engaged in the P&M Asian subseries primarily are conducting normative Confucian studies, they need, on the one hand, to comprehend its underlying values, principles, and perspectives from the inside, and on the other hand, to maintain a critical stance, employing rigorous analysis and avoiding undue ethnocentrism.

[2] The majority of volumes within the P&M subseries focus on bioethical and healthcare issues in East Asian societies, examining them through a Confucian lens. However, it is important to acknowledge that while Confucianism is a prominent cultural force in these societies, other religions and cultures, such as Buddhism and Daoism, are also present and influential.

as well the 74th P&M volume titled *Bioethics and Moral Content: National Traditions of Health Care Morality* edited by Tris Engelhardt and Lisa Rasmussen (2002). Both appeared within the subseries "Asian Studies in Bioethics and the Philosophy of Medicine" via Kluwer Academic Publishers. In subsequent years, Asian or Asian-based researchers became increasingly engaged in this work. This process eventually turned East Asian bioethics from a vision to a committed and feasible reality embodied in the subsequent publications of the series since the 21st century. The subseries in this regard suggests a truly global movement in the community of bioethics and the philosophy of medicine. It triggers responses not only from the center of the global ethics community, namely the West (Walker 2009; Sullivan 2016; Pennings and Symons 2024), but also from non-Western, notably Asian countries (Elliott et al. 2010), which play an important role in determining its course.

Unsurprisingly, a sense of the challenge can only be gained from looking into the volumes themselves, which include not only well-thought-out arguments on perennial hard problems in bioethics but also fresh questions enabled by the introduction of alternative views. Central to this approach is the role of the family in East Asian bioethics. In this article, we focus on the theme of the place of the family in East Asian bioethics and review the volumes and authors in the associated subseries.

9.2 A Family-Based Approach to Bioethics

9.2.1 Thinking About Bioethics Comparatively

Moral diversity is a lived reality. Moral visions, regardless of the situation, may lapse into error not only in the realm of philosophical analysis, but even in that of life and morals. There are increasingly more bioethical issues whose resolution requires not only a full appreciation of moral diversity at the global level, but, more importantly, an even deeper exploration of the potential of cultural and religious resources at the local level. In the first few years of the 21st century, the publication of three volumes marked the beginning of a new phase in bioethics in East Asian societies. These volumes include *Confucian Bioethics* (no. 61 of the P&M series, 1999); *Cross-Cultural Perspectives on the (Im)Possibility of Global Bioethics* edited by Julia Tao Lai Po-wah (no. 71 of the P&M series 2002); and *Bioethics: Asian Perspectives. A Quest for Moral Diversity* edited by Ren-Zong Qiu (no. 80 of the P&M series, 2004).

A sure sign of the early fledging movement of East Asian bioethics is the 2002 volume *Cross-Cultural Perspectives on the (Im)Possibility of Global Bioethics*. As the title suggests, awareness of moral diversity has developed to meet the conceptual and practical challenges of bioethics. The volume features an expanded vision on several fronts. First, the contributors of the volume are from diverse cultural – Hong Kong, Taiwan, mainland China, Japan, Germany, and the U.S. – as well as religious backgrounds, varying from orthodox Christian to secular liberal egalitarian to Confucian perspectives. The second feature is the volume's diversified content. As well as a theoretical analysis that provides the philosophical basis for bioethical disputes and healthcare policy, discussions on a wide range of contentious topics are included, such as sex reassignment surgery, prenatal genetic screening or treatment, and genetic engineering.

Nevertheless, the most attractive aspect of Tao's volume is the challenge it poses to the universalistic view that is centered on the idea of individual liberty. In this view, the handling of moral issues is based on the principle that individuals have the right to make decisions on their own, which should and must be respected by others and guaranteed by institutional and governmental policies. This entails practices such as individual-oriented informed consent, which is regarded as the standard practice for decision-making in healthcare. According to this individualistic model, global bioethics inherently possesses a cosmopolitan characteristic that prioritizes the moral agency of individuals over the communal structures based on kinship, personal relationships, ethnicity, or religious affiliations in healthcare policy. The contributors to the volume propose that readers expand their perspective beyond the confines of the current Western framework. More specifically, a significant differentiation is made between the individualistic notion of autonomy, which has traditionally been regarded as progressive and universal, and a revitalized, culturally sensitive, and pluralistic moral understanding presented in the volume. This viewpoint necessitates that bioethicists familiarize themselves with the vast diversity in lifestyles and perspectives. According to some authors for this volume, the issue with Western bioethics lies in its transformation into a cosmopolitan myth, despite its inherent cultural and ideological specificity.

Published in 2004, *Bioethics: Asian Perspectives. A Quest for Moral Diversity* provides further evidence that a general turn had already begun. A noteworthy feature of the volume is a manifest quest for a cultural identity, which was referred to as the introduction of "Asian perspectives" in bioethics, or, succinctly, Asian bioethics. The main argument, according to Qiu, is against an "overarching universal ethics or global ethics" even though some values might be shared among cultures. Emphasis, correspondingly, was placed on the demonstration of the diversity in moral visions, moral reasoning, and above all moral identities. In this matter, consideration of the variety of authorship is important. Qiu stresses that the authorship of the volume consists mostly of non-Western contributors – from mainland China, Hong Kong, Japan, South Korea, the Philippines, and Nepal – as well as researchers who are of Chinese origin and work at universities in North America. This may suggest an attempt to construct an identity grounded in the East–West binary opposition.

However, it could be critiqued that the argument presented for "Asian bioethics" in this volume lacks clarity in supporting a radical change in the field of bioethics. Firstly, the term "Asian bioethics" is often used interchangeably with "Chinese" or "Confucian" bioethics without adequate explanation in the volume. This approach may obscure the internal cultural, religious, and linguistic diversity within Asia or East Asia, which extends beyond a mere geographic expression or a vague construct with a Sinocentric bias. Secondly, similar to Tao's volume, Qiu's volume covers a wide range of topics, including cloning, brain death, euthanasia, birth control, HIV/

AIDS, and healthcare systems. However, certain arguments presented in the volume, such as the defense of China's former one-child policy, have become outdated and irrelevant due to the significant changes in China's population policy over the past two decades. Thirdly, while the "global versus local" dichotomy proposed by Qiu is thought-provoking and somewhat reasonable, relying on stereotypical depictions of "the West" hampers the understanding of the underlying systems of "Western bioethics" and the biomedical and ethical contexts associated with it. Creating new generalizations around the issue of anti-universalism can be equally concerning as the previous Eurocentric approach taken in bioethics.

It is not surprising that a more focused volume would be better equipped to address concerns regarding Confucian biomedical morality and its practical applications. *Confucian Bioethics*, edited by Fan, appears to have aimed at concentrating solely on Confucian ethical perspectives in response to contemporary bioethical challenges and the growing demand for particularity or specificity in bioethics. Notably, the contributors to this volume were all Chinese scholars studying or working in North America, possessing familiarity with modern Western ethical theories alongside their adherence to the Confucian way of life. This unique combination allows for a more compelling and targeted exploration of bioethical issues associated with the Chinese people and the well-defined tradition of Confucianism. Consequently, it becomes easier to compare the Confucian perspective on bioethical matters with the universal claims of global bioethics, which often assert justification based solely on reason and apply indiscriminately to all individuals and societies. In the vision presented by the authors in this volume, the latter perspective may reveal more about modern Western liberalism, which represents just one among many viewpoints, rather than true cosmopolitanism.

The advent of a workable conceptual framework also meets a need for an identity in the Geertzian sense. In East Asian societies, such as mainland China, Hong Kong, Taiwan, Japan, and South Korea, Confucian values, notably the importance attached to the family, still play a role in both conventional moral and political life. This is where the distinction between a "real" Confucian bioethics instead of what Fan refers to as "museum" Confucianism was made: traditions, if viewed as a repository for more than inanimate objects or a sense of previous occupation, could produce a meaningful transformation in the image of bioethics that holds sway in contemporary academia. Moreover, an enhanced moral vision that incorporates the respect and goodwill of bioethics towards existing moral diversity has the potential to foster a program or guide to action – whether legal or political – rather than an armchair analysis for its own sake. The subsequent volumes of the subseries over the past two decades have demonstrated the growing significance of Confucian bioethics as a prominent voice among diverse perspectives in the global arena of bioethics. What began as an idea in the 1999 volume has evolved into a substantial and influential presence, solidifying its position within the field.

9.2.2 *Clinical Decision Making: Informed Consent, Trust, and Other Issues*

Philosophical thinking about an alternative approach to bioethics leads to discussions on more specific topics at the clinical, institutional, and even disciplinary levels. It opens dialogue on topics ranging from medical decision-making or informed consent, to the politics of healthcare. The contributions of the Asian subseries in this regard include, in chronological order, *The Family, Medical Decision-Making, and Biotechnology* (2007), edited by Shui Chuen Lee, *China: Bioethics, Trust, and the Challenge of the Market* (2007), edited by Julia Tao, and *Family-oriented Informed Consent: East Asian and American Perspectives* (2015), edited by Ruiping Fan.

A rough outline for the application of a Confucian approach to contemporary bioethical issues can be found in *The Family, Medical Decision-Making, and Biotechnology*, which was edited by Shui Chuen Lee and presented as the 91st volume of the "Philosophy and Medicine" series in 2007. The volume consists of articles from theoretical and empirical perspectives. The first perspective involves a philosophical exposition of the family's centrality in Confucian thought as well as its ethical and ontological significance. Discussions on topics that later became both widely known and vividly disputed in the East Asian bioethical community – such as the Confucian understanding of decision-making or truth-telling in the healthcare context – were integrated into the volume; the second focuses on the challenges that emerging technologies pose to the Confucian tradition (to be discussed in Sect. 2.3).

In 2015, a significant contribution to the discourse on informed consent was made with the publication of "Family-oriented Informed Consent: East Asian and American Perspectives." This volume presents several compelling arguments in favor of family-oriented informed consent. While individual-based informed consent remains the prevailing norm in Western cultures and has been adopted or adapted by non-Western cultures, this volume uniquely benefits from the insights of four American contributors and 14 Asian contributors from Hong Kong, mainland China, South Korea, and Taiwan. In the United States, individual-directed informed consent is enforced through legislation such as the Health Insurance Portability and Accountability Act (HIPAA) within contemporary biomedical practices. However, alternative approaches to safeguarding and promoting well-being receive limited attention within the Western-dominated bioethics community. Recognizing the family as a foundational concept, the volume proposes the adoption of a family-oriented model of informed consent specifically within the context of East Asian healthcare. While the family-oriented model of informed consent may face objections, such as concerns about respecting individual wishes or interests, the authors in this volume endeavor to defend its legitimacy within the framework of East Asian biomedical practices characterized by prominent Confucian moral and cultural influences. Regardless of their success or failure, these attempts provide valuable academic resources for further study and contemplation.

On a conceptual level, a major difference exists between the broad and strict meanings of the family. Discussions surrounding biomedical decision-making in post-industrial Western societies often revolve around the concept of the family as a voluntary social entity, irrespective of its structure or the sexual orientation of its members. However, for most researchers from East Asian societies, the concept of the family was largely understood to be of the "traditional" type, which was built around a heterosexual couple and which usually involves three generations - the couple, their children, and their respective parents. While the premise concerning the "strict" or "traditional" family as many Asian researcher see it, has a factual basis, it was also endowed with a normative connotation. That is, the engagement of family members in informed consent, which is critical to medical decision-making, is deemed not only a reality in a Confucian cultural context but, more importantly, as morally acceptable or even appropriate and just.

The focus of this volume is to examine the limitations of applying the individualistic approach of the Western medical establishment and social decision-making apparatus to the Confucian context of East Asian biomedical practices. It presents an alternative model for more balanced decision-making in these practices. The primary concern with informed consent arises from the shortcomings of the individualistic model. In contemporary Western biomedical practices, informed consent predominantly relies on an autonomous individualist perspective. The family is often viewed as potentially conflicting with the ideal of personal autonomy, which is considered a fundamental principle of equality and social justice, particularly within the liberal tradition. It should be noted that the purpose of the US/Western system is to allow patients to decide whether or not to involve their families, rather than preventing them from seeking advice from their loved ones. Many families do engage in regular conversations about healthcare decisions. However, under the Western model, the patient ultimately holds the final decision-making power or authority, whereas the Confucian model emphasizes shared power or authority between the patient and the family. In Western biomedical institutions, the decision of whether the family should be involved in the decision-making process is typically left to the patient, following a documented procedure. While this does not discourage family involvement institutionally, it places individual decisions as a primary requirement and positions them at the core of informed consent. As a result, patients are expected or even encouraged to make decisions independently.

The emphasis on individual decisions in informed consent has multiple drawbacks, as elaborated by several contributors to the volume. Firstly, it is important to note that the individualistic approach may not necessarily facilitate optimal decision-making for the individual. According to Jue Wang's chapter in the volume, a Confucian perspective suggests that optimal decisions can only be achieved through practical reasoning rooted in the practice of family interdependence. This perspective emphasizes the importance of reaching out to others rather than isolating oneself, as it promotes a deeper understanding of the complexities involved in decision-making. As Jue Wang shows, the critically ill can become estranged from others and deviate from the proper direction that they need to truly follow because of the influence of diseases or disorders. They may only return with the help of the communities to which they belong, which can be interpreted as an extension of their families, or in many cases, the family per se. Individualized informed consent, as she argues, depends on a fundamentally flawed and narrow understanding of individual autonomy. Second, the patient's capability to exercise the right to self-determination is overrated in high-tech medical circumstances, such as the Intensive Care Unit (ICU). In fact, it would be unrealistic to assume a clearcut dividing line between seeking aggressive medical intervention and simply ending such intervention, given the increasingly formidable power of life-support equipment in biomedicine. Third, individualized informed consent does not conform to the cultural reality of East Asian societies, especially when it comes to medical decisions. For instance, reports from both South Korea and Taiwan show that family involvement in personal decisions, notably regarding medical issues, is common. Finally, the principle that sustains the individual-oriented model of informed consent can result in insensitivity or even indifference to the complexities of medical practices.

In contrast, according to some contributors of the volume, family-oriented informed consent can be devised to circumvent the negative consequences of individualism's failure concerning neglected families and moral plights. The justification of family-oriented informed consent corresponds, on a descriptive level, to the socio-cultural fact that the family in its "traditional" forms is a fundamental unit for making medical decisions for the patient in East Asian societies. On a normative level, the family-oriented model of informed consent, or broadly, decision-making, can be justified in four ways. First, family involvement in medical decision-making can help alleviate the stress caused by the dehumanizing proclivities of biomedicine and provide care and emotional support for patients. Second, the family has both good knowledge of its members' physical and mental needs to make better decisions and the ability to implement the decisions that are taken. Third, family involvement in informed consent would yield better medical outcomes in difficult cases, such as cadaveric organ donation or participation in clinical trials. Finally, the family's engagement in medical decisions is supported by Confucian moral virtues and the ontological-metaphysical account of the family – both of which are still prevalent in East Asian societies. Similar to Christianity, according to Engelhardt (2013), the family under the Confucian account is appreciated as a deep, normative social entity that carries both ethical and ontological significance. The corollary of the Confucian metaphysics of the family is that the flourishing of the family precedes human flourishing, and is a prerequisite for the latter.

However, this does not imply that family-oriented informed consent is without its challenges in the modern world. Among the most representative challenges are concerns that the family may ignore or override the individual and damage the interests of the latter by imposing a kind of family paternalism. Other relevant challenges in a similar vein include issues of truth-telling to patients and preparing advance directives before the patient has no or limited civil capacity. Although exact ways to meet these challenges require thorough discussion, according to Fan, Jue Wang, Wenqing Zhao, and many other contributors to the volume, the key to a solution is the standard by which medical decisions are taken, be they taken in a family- or individual-oriented manner. The family and the individual are not necessarily antagonistic. The Confucian approach to bioethics does not rest on a utilitarian basis providing for the calculation of benefits and costs. Nor is it intended to provide a fixed formula that fits all contexts. Instead, it recommends fair consent solutions that are structured under the guidance of virtues in interested parties and are fundamentally contextual.

Concerns about the healthcare system date to the beginning of the East Asian bioethical movement. During the first decade of the 21st century, widespread discontent regarding healthcare provision among Chinese people attracted increasing attention. Soaring costs combined with explosive growth in the number of reports of bribery, malpractice, and medical disputes sparked heated discussion about the direction of China's healthcare reform and what path it should take. Discussions on social justice in healthcare in relation to the Confucian tradition can be dated to the 1999 volume *Confucian Bioethics* and culminated in 2007, when two volumes of the Asian subseries were published, both of which contributed to sustained discussions. Three articles included in the 2007 volume *The Family, Medical Decision-Making, and Biotechnology* focus on the problem of healthcare, rationing, and responsibility, using the examples of Singapore and Hong Kong, both of which exist in an "in-between" position between the East and West.

At the same time, the 96th volume of the P&M series, *Bioethics, Trust, and the Challenge of the Market* edited by Julia Tao (2008), is a whole volume dedicated to China's healthcare crisis and attempts to give advice on how to rebuild China's beleaguered healthcare system. Although healthcare policy is known to present moral and political challenges worldwide, the situation in contemporary China is distinctive in that its healthcare reform is complex and interwoven with the political and economic transformation marked by the policy of reform and opening-up implemented since the late 1970s.

In general, the volume distinguishes between three approaches to healthcare policy: (1) the Western social-democratic welfare approach, which is based on a social welfare ideology and committed to equal access to basic healthcare for all members of society; (2) the Singaporean approach, which is marked by mandatory family health saving accounts; and (3) a market-based approach, which, some suggest, would be a solution to China's disturbingly disoriented healthcare reform. However, each approach has strengths and weaknesses. The social-democratic approach adopted by most European countries and Canada has proven to pose a severe financial burden on the social-welfare state and could hurt China's economy. This could be a fatal flaw for a country with a large poor population and stifle its economic future, which is crucial for the legitimacy of the Party-state. Alternatively, a market solution to China's healthcare crisis has much allure, especially regarding the country's transition to a market economy. However, embracing the free market is likely to pose a challenge to the official socialist agenda and draw the government into a damaging ideological mire in which its credentials will also be on trial. Given the situation, following the Singaporean model was once regarded as a promising option. The model puts some weight on the health responsibility of the family through financial instruments while at the same time leaving individuals and families with healthcare choices. Moreover, such a model is thought to be a successful integration of Confucian moral traditions into the healthcare system and could guide an East Asian approach to healthcare policy.

Thus, to what extent and in what ways China's healthcare reform can learn from Singapore, and sometimes Hong Kong, the situation of which is somewhat analogous to Singapore, forms the center of attention throughout the volume. Overall, contributors to the volume agree that the market is not a panacea; unregulated markets favoring private institutions, typically for-profit ones, tend to produce undesirable results. According to the contributors, a mix of public–private health care provision and the corresponding distribution of health responsibility between the family and the state implemented by Singapore strikes a better balance between social benefits and efficiency. Some Chinese contributors have examined contemporary Chinese healthcare policy, notably its evolution and its realized and unrealized moral commitments. Nevertheless, the majority of the volume includes normative analyses of how efficient and sustainable healthcare provision can be attained in alignment with Confucian heritage, in which the family plays a central role. More specifically, China's difficult changes in healthcare policy should be seen as a call to restore trust, as suggested by Tao, and to change the way of thinking. Confucian values can be a resource to foster not only the benevolence of the physician but also institutional integrity (Iltis) or a culture of responsibility (Fransen). Furthermore, as Fan puts it, from a Confucian perspective, the idea of welfare is essentially family-centered and not built upon an egalitarian underpinning. This provides an alternative framework with which a top-level design of the national healthcare system that is more suitable for China can be developed. At the same time, to engage in discussion also gives new life to Confucian thought and creates what Fan calls "reconstructionist Confucianism."

9.2.3 Biotechnologies

The moral consequences of biotechnology in relation to multiculturalism have attracted the attention of bioethicists since at least 2007, as shown in *The Family, Medical Decision-Making, and Biotechnology* edited by Shui Chuen Lee (2007). Seven (Chapters 7, 9, and 10, 11, 12, 13, 14) of the 17 articles included in the collection focus on the application of emerging biotechnologies from a broad theoretical or comparative perspective: sex selection technology, organ donation, and human embryonic stem cell research. Although, like in mainland China, sex selection is banned in Taiwan, ethical analysis shows that the preference for boys, or sexism more generally, is entrenched in societies deeply shaped by Confucian thought, and requires more careful consideration in legislation to protect women's well-being and reproductive autonomy. Comparative studies of research policies in different societies have revealed curious discrepancies. Unlike Western societies, East Asian societies tend to adopt more permissive approaches to embryo research. While some researcher put this down to "Western liberal individualism" (Fan), some others argue for the influence of Judeo-Christian theological ethics (Engelhardt), including the Islamic approach of Near Asian countries reported by Aksoy et al., on Western thinking about embryo research.

The growing interest in cultural influences on organ donation among Asian and Asian-based bioethicists, particularly the role that the family plays, later developed into an entire collection dedicated to the topic. In the latest volume of the subseries published in 2023, *Incentives and Disincentives in Organ Donation: a multicultural study among Beijing, Chicago, Tehran and Hong Kong* edited by Ruiping Fan (2023), researchers focus on the moral and cultural dimensions involved in the application of the biotechnology of organ transplantation. While patients in need benefit greatly from organ transplantation, organ shortages are common in both living and cadaveric donations worldwide. This necessitates examination of incentive and disincentive models, as well as of how organ donation rates are conditioned by cultural factors. Generally, incentive models can be divided into three types: liberal (honorary), compensationalist, and familist. The liberal or honorary model, which was adopted in North America and most European countries, presupposes that the action of donating one's organ is driven by altruistic and egalitarian motives and can be encouraged through measures designed for honorary incentives such as medals or thank you notes. In contrast, the compensationalist model emphasizes the financial compensation provided to the donor. As shown in the Islamic Republic of Iran, such compensation is not given by the recipient but endowed by the government in monetary or non-monetary (e.g., health insurance) forms to hedge the risk of organ trafficking. The familist model for organ donation, first devised by Israel, prioritizes family members of donors and incorporates a corresponding stratified priority system for family beneficiaries. The national system for the distribution of donated organs established in mainland China in the 2000s primarily follows the familist model, suggesting the importance the Chinese assign to the family.

Benefiting from authors from four societies – namely, mainland China (taking Beijing as a sample), Hong Kong, Iran (Tehran as the sample), and the United States (Chicago as the sample) – the collection celebrates a curious multicultural perspective in analyzing moral considerations and policy design regarding the improvement of organ donation rates. The collection provides a varied and well-balanced account of the incentive problem at individual, societal, and cultural levels. The combined use of empirical studies (notably quantitative analysis and extensive in-depth interviews with donors, recipients, family members, medical professionals, policymakers, and ethicists with different cultural backgrounds), literature reviews, and theoretical analyses makes the collection's arguments organized and plausible. Examinations of incentives and relevant public perceptions in the four societies suggest significant differences in incentives and disincentives between societies.

Of particular interest is that the family's impact on organ donation may have both positive and negative consequences, depending on the family's social and cultural milieu. For example, the idea of appropriate death, notably concerns over bodily integrity even in death, can constitute an obstacle to organ donation, as the biotechnology of organ transplantation entails the removal of the donor's organ(s), typically within a specific time limit. This partly explains the considerably low donation rates in mainland China and Hong Kong, both of which have culturally entrenched legacy values placed on filial piety and encounter difficulties with deceased organ donations. A package of incentives or mixed incentive measures, rather than deploying a single incentive model, has been suggested to be ethically justifiable, politically legitimate, and more likely to improve donation rates. Sufficient thought given to the discrepancies in cultural and social values, as convincingly shown throughout the 16 articles, is key to optimizing mixed incentive measures.

Moreover, while a Hong Kong-based survey suggests that the vast majority of the Hong Kong public approves familist incentives such as offering a columbarium niche to a deceased donor, there are also concerns about whether it would inappropriately favor large families while putting those with fewer siblings or children – the number of these people is increasing in the process of urbanization – in a disadvantaged position. Moreover, families may have different ideas regarding organ donation. In extreme cases, this leads to potentially compelling donation against a deceased family member's wish or, conversely, the family's veto of a deceased member's donation wishes. Given this situation, a family's wishes can conflict with an individual's will and undermine individual autonomy. A defense by Fan, the editor of the collection, for the "familist decision model" in organ donation is that concerns about impairing individual autonomy can be regarded as a reflection of an individualistic mentality, which, however, may be problematic from a family-based Confucian perspective. An agreement within the family regarding organ donation wishes is recommended prior to possible disagreements that may emerge between the individual and his or her family while living or posthumously.

9.3 Challenges and Further Explorations

The transformation from a traditional to an industrialized society led to the breakdown of the family clan and the rise of modern individuals in China throughout the 20th century. The predominant Chinese ideology has no longer been Confucianism since the establishment of the People of Republic China in 1949. The trend towards individualization was sped up due to China's turn to a market economy and untied its Communist ideological control since the late 1970s. Nevertheless, the Chinese society has undergone massive changes since the beginning of the 21st century. Far from being overwhelmed by an apparently increasingly strong individualist consciousness in younger generations, the power of the family was sometimes strengthened by the way it functions in realignment with these trends (Yan 2021; Jing 2000).

The relevance of Confucianism, or tradition broadly, to the contemporary world can only be properly understood in this context. While some observers have noticed this intriguing realignment, philosophers and ethicists to date seem to have paid insufficient attention.[3] A closer and updated examination of contemporary Chinese society, in particular, and Asian societies in general, can provide more insight into the understanding of bioethical issues.

[3] A few Chinese philosophers have made exceptional strides in their recent research, exploring the contrasting features of Confucian culture's familist orientation and the individualist culture prevalent in the modern Western context. See Yang (2017), Zhang (2017) and Sun (2019).

Another issue that calls for further exploration is cultural and religious differences within and across East Asian societies. Although some of the authors or editors of the subseries have long recognized this, much needs to be done to tap into the full potential of a diversified, well-communicated rather than narrow-minded East Asian ethos. A full evaluation of the complexities of us–them negotiations, which are represented in both intercultural and intracultural communications, will be of great help to future bioethics.

9.4 Conclusion

As convincingly revealed by the growing number of volumes in the Asian subseries, an increased awareness of moral diversity in bioethics is not only feasible but also imperative because of political, economic, and moral crises caused by the elevated global state of conflict. This subseries is successful in delineating what happens when global bioethical ideas and practices diffuse into the cultural and institutional contexts of East Asian societies, which are deeply influenced by Confucian perspectives on the family, social justice, and morality. Benefiting from the contributors who engage in and enact an East-West dialogue, the subseries tells a broad story of how the global can settle down and made local, as well as how the local can be navigated to generate global impact and eventually become global.

Acknowledgments We express our gratitude to Lisa M. Rasmussen for her meticulous and comprehensive feedback on the previous version of this essay. Her valuable comments have greatly contributed to enhancing our discussions and shaping the final version of the essay. The research leading to this essay received funding from the National Social Science Foundation of China (NSSFC) (Grant No. 23BZX052).

References

Elliott, J. M., W. C. Ho, and S. S. N. Lim, eds. 2010. *Bioethics in Singapore: The Ethical Microcosm*. World Scientific Publishing Co. Pte. Ltd.

Engelhardt, H. T., Jr. 2013. The Family: Crucial to and Divisive in Bioethics. *International Journal of Chinese & Comparative Philosophy of Medicine* 11 (2): 113–127.

Engelhardt, H. T., and L. M. Rasmussen, eds. 2002. *Bioethics and Moral Content: National Traditions of Health Care Morality-Papers Dedicated in Tribute to Kazumasa Hoshino*. Dordrecht: Springer.

Fan, R., ed. 1999. *Confucian Bioethics*. Dordrecht: Kluwer Academic Publishers.

Fan, R., ed. 2015. *Family-Oriented Informed Consent East Asian and American Perspectives*. Dordrecht: Springer.

Fan, R., ed. 2023. *Incentives and Disincentives in Organ Donation: A Multicultural Study Among Beijing, Chicago, Tehran and Hong Kong*. Cham, Switzerland: Springer.

Geertz, C. 1988. *Works and Lives: The Anthropologist as Author*. Stanford, CA: Stanford University Press.

Jing, J. 2000. *Feeding China's Little Emperors: Food, Children, and Social Change*. Stanford, CA: Stanford University Press.

Lee, S. C., ed. 2007. *The Family, Medical Decision-Making, and Biotechnology: Critical Reflections on Asian Moral Perspectives*. Dordrecht: Springer.

Pennings, S., and X. Symons. 2024. First Among Equals? Adaptive Preferences and the Limits of Autonomy in Medical Ethics. *Journal of Medical Ethics* 50:212–218.

Qiu, R., ed. 2004. *Bioethics: Asian Perspectives: A Quest For Moral Diversity*. Dordrecht: Springer.

Sullivan, L. S. 2016. Uncovering Metaethical Assumptions in Bioethical Discourse across Cultures. *Kennedy Institute of Ethics Journal* 26 (1): 47–78. https://doi.org/10.1353/ken.2016.0003.

Sun, X., and 孙向晨. 2019. *On the Family: Individuals and Relatives* 论家:个体与亲亲. Shanghai: Huadong Normal University Press.

Tao Lai Po-wah, J., ed. 2002. *Cross-Cultural Perspectives on the (im)Possibility of Global Bioethics*. Dordrecht: Springer.

Tao Lai Po-wah, J., ed. 2008. *China: Bioethics, Trust, and the Challenge of the Market*. Dordrecht: Springer.

Walker, T. 2009. What Principlism Misses. *Journal of Medical Ethics* 35 (2): 29–231.

Yan, Y. 2021. *Chinese Families Upside Down: Intergenerational Dynamics and Neo-Familism in the Early 21st Century*. Boston: Brill academic publication.

Yang, X., and 杨效思. 2017. *Philosophy of the Family: The Blind Spot of the West* 家哲学:西方的盲点. Beijing: Shangwu Press.

Zhang, X., and 张祥龙. 2017. *Family and Filiality: From Eastern and Western Perspectives* 家与孝:从中西视野看. Beijing: Sanlian Books.

Part III
Topics—Selected Topics and Reprints from the Series' History

Chapter 10
Lost in Translation: How 1979 Proved Pivotal for Bioethics and Why We Need a Narrative Account of Morality in Medicine

D. Micah Hester

A ten-year span, between 1969 and 1979, was all it took to establish the foundations of modern bioethics. In '69 and '70, the Hasting Center, the Kennedy Institute of Ethics, and Penn State-Hershey's medical humanities program identified bioethics as an academic, scholarly endeavor. By 1973 the National Commission manifested? Governmental interests in ethics and medicine. Court cases arising from clinical situations like the 1976 case of Karen Ann Quinlan spoke to the idea that hospitals should establish institutional bodies that can think through ethically challenging situations.

As a nascent but growing academic "demi-discipline" (cf Jonsen 1997), bioethics in the '70s needed a carefully considered base of scholarship in order to ground itself as a legitimate intellectual, professional enterprise. While books and articles had appeared in the decades before (e.g., Fletcher 1954), those works identified a "gap" in our moral considerations about medicine and science, stimulating others to more comprehensive and detailed discussions. In fact, the book series, Philosophy and Medicine, itself, was established by Tris Engelhardt and Stuart Spicker in 1975 precisely to "examine the conceptual background in terms of which questions in medical ethics can best be assayed," building a scholarly foundation for the field of bioethics. But what eluded the field was a *lingua franca*—a common language—that could ground moral insights and debates under the disciplinary umbrella known as "bioethics."

By the end of this pivotal decade all that changed with the publication of two critical manuscripts, *The Belmont Report* (1978) and the *Principles of Biomedical Ethics* (1979). These two documents suggested that a fundamental, limited set of ethical norms of practice could be identified for both the research and clinical

D. M. Hester (✉)
Department of Medical Humanities & Bioethics, UAMS, Little Rock, AR, USA
e-mail: DMHester@uams.edu

L. M. Rasmussen, S. Holm (eds.), *50 Years of Philosophy and Medicine*,
Philosophy and Medicine 150, https://doi.org/10.1007/978-3-031-95175-6_10

environments, norms that spoke to the obligations of investigators and providers, respectively. These basic "principles" of research (respect for persons, beneficence, justice) and biomedical ([respect for] autonomy, beneficence, nonmaleficence, justice) ethics capture important aspects of moral truth in medicine and were quickly adopted by bioethicist and clinicians/investigators, alike.

To be sure, the principle-based approach was not without its vocal detractors early on, but even in the face of strong critiques, so-called "principlism" increased in usage through both scholarship and education. Fast forwarding nearly 50 years later, there is hardly any healthcare professional, trainee, student who has not heard about the 3–4 basic bioethical principles, and nearly every issue of a professional journal that has an article on ethics in medicine in it will allude at some point to the principles (whether as set and unquestioned or as problematic and concerning).

In light of this background, the focus of this chapter, while recognizing the importance of our established biomedical principles, turns to what was and is lost when reducing the moral framework of medicine to said-principles.[1] The problem is, in part, that a robust discussion and awareness of various philosophies of medicine have receded while more targeted use of basic (and often "sloganized") norms are asked to do more than they were intended to do. I will demonstrate this by focusing on two essays on clinical judgment published the same year (1979) as the first edition of *The Principles…*—essays written for the 6th volume of the series Philosophy and Medicine (also published in 1979), not by humanities scholars but by erudite, practicing physicians, Edmund Pellegrino and Eric Cassell. I will suggest that while we remain well-served by careful elucidation and nuanced application of ethical principles in medicine, taking a step back to consider larger frameworks for understanding the "art and science" of medicine can substantively and positively affect the ethics of medicine, as well.

In the late 1990s, during his presidential address to the Society for Health and Human Values, Al Jonsen muses, "Many of us have wondered how the desiccated moral philosophy of the 1960s turned into the vigorous ethics of bioethics…" (Jonsen 1997). While Joseph Fletcher's 1954 work, *Medicine and Morals*, made an early statement about the need for a discussion of the ethics of healthcare, the rise of analytic philosophy in the United States had pushed aside value theory and moral philosophy in many corners of academia. As such, we found, as Tom Beauchamp notes, "Prior to the early 1970s, there was no firm ground in which a commitment to principles or even ethical theory could take root in biomedical ethics" (35, 2010). Stemming from their collaborations at the Kennedy Institute of Ethics, Beauchamp and his colleague, James Childress, endeavored to effect change in bioethics to give "the embryonic field of bioethics a shared method for attacking its problems,…[with] some minimal coherence and uniformity" (36, 2010). Akin to what *The Belmont Report* (1978) did for research, Beauchamp and Childress identified fundamental ethical norms in *clinical* care. And so in 1979, they published the first edition of a

[1] For accounts of various "losses" in the history of bioethics, cf. Baker (2024) and Evans (2012).

singularly important text in the field, *Principles of Biomedical Ethics*. It is this work that elucidates four basic ethical principles, or "action guides," for clinical practice in medicine.

Much has been written in bioethics both about and with the principles, and it is not my intention here to recount myriad uses and debates. Whatever one's thoughts are on these principles—whether championed as "basic" and "fundamental" or couched (somewhat deridingly) as "principlism" or "The Georgetown Mantra"—it seems that one important reason for their rapid and steadfast acceptance in the field is that "Principles were used to present frameworks of evaluative assumptions so that they could be used by, and readily understood by, people with many different forms of professional training. The distilled morality found in principles gave people a shared and serviceable group of general norms for analyzing many types of moral problems" (36, 2010). As sociologist John Evans puts it, "Principlism created a set of predetermined ends, portrayed as universally held by people. [With this, t]he bioethics profession....now had solid jurisdiction over research bioethics and health-care ethics consultation" (Evans 2012, 68).

In other words, it is no overstatement to say that the principles-approach of Beauchamp and Childress flourished after the publication of the first edition. Again, whatever one's take, it is hard to deny that the principles capture important aspects of moral truth—that individuals matter, that their well-being matters, that fairness matters. The principles speak to these moral issues, even if we may not all agree they do so in a satisfying, robust, clear way. By speaking to these issues, though, they found fertile soil in which to take root. In fact, they remain today the most cited framework for bioethical deliberation, taught in medical schools and other health professional training, used in licensure exams for health professions, and continually applied or debated throughout the medical ethics literature. A simple search in Google Scholar or PubMed will readily find articles and books published just within the last couple of years that either refer to the principles in support of some ethical analysis of clinical care or take the principles as the main foil in order to argue some other ethical insight or framework.

My point is that, for better or worse, principles *did become* that *lingua franca* for bioethics—language that when doing the work of bioethics we all must either use or explain why we are not. But the use (and abuse) of this framework as well as its ubiquity has created a culture of bioethics in practice that regularly relies on *expressing* the principles to others rather than *understanding* them robustly. They have become slogans, even caricatures, not so much "readily understood by" the clinician who expresses them, as merely stated and broadly agreed to. Of course, this problem is not to be laid fully at the feet of Beauchamp and Childress themselves, but they are also not wholly without some blame.

Initially more concerned with the role of moral theory in relationship to professional practice, Beauchamp and Childress describe their principles in early editions as norms that arise from a "convergence" of deontological and utilitarian considerations (through such thinkers a WD Ross and William Frankena). Here, then, the authors claim a theoretical basis, but a fairly tenuous one where traditionally competing philosophical frameworks are taken not as divergent but instead as co-foundations of one and the same set of principles. This tenuousness is evident in the first edition when the concept of autonomy vacillates between "freedom of action" (a la Mill) and "freedom of will" (a la Kant), shifts that are sure to raise the hackles of many moral philosophers. This vacillation leads to their "principle of autonomy" (as it was then known) being explicated primarily by a lengthy discussion to the importance and practice of "informed consent" rather than a careful rendering of a consistent account of autonomy, itself (1979, 62–85). Eventually, then, Beauchamp and Childress (from the 4th edition onward) unshackle the principles from any particular moral philosophy or theoretical basis, rooted instead in "the common morality" and described as "pre-theoretical" principles that can find reasoned justification from a wide variety of moral theories—a kind of Rawlsian "overlapping consensus" among a number of comprehensive moral doctrines. In fact, with principles grounded in common morality, what results is that *theories* that do not comport with the principles are themselves to be considered prima facie morally suspicious.

To be clear, neither Beauchamp nor Childress eschew the place of theory in ethical reasoning. In fact, it is clear in their own individual work that they both hold tightly to particular moral philosophies. However, as a form of "applied ethics," they suggest that their principle-based approach is best understood at the level of the principles themselves, and not in relation to any particular moral theory. Of course, this is, in part, why they have been so successful, creating a kind of "big tent" approach to practical ethics that attempts to forestall theoretical debates in order to get significant everyday moral work done. And yet, as I have argued elsewhere (Hester 2001), no moral norms can stand outside of theory entirely—they involve commitments to intentions or consequences or virtues (or some combination). They implicate claims about human nature(s), the moral life, and the philosophy and practice of medicine that should not go unrecognized but instead, once recognized, become the fodder for discussion and debate about both the acceptability and usefulness for the principles themselves. And while there may be convergence in the common morality and among ethical theories about these principles, any supposed convergence stands at such a high level of abstraction that it leaves the principles themselves almost completely unfettered and open to a variety of interpretations and uses, undermining their place as a truly *common* language. For instance, the utilitarian suggests the importance of "autonomy of action," while the deontologist leans into "autonomy of will"—the former looking to see what actions can be allowed or curtailed while the latter addressing a conditional state for the possibility of moral activity in the first place.

Again, my point here is not to adjudicate the promises and challenges of principles but to note that they set a particular kind of moral culture in medicine, a culture that is less concerned with what *grounds* our moral consideration (save, maybe, for common morality), and more concerned with how to *frame* moral issues. Framing delimits but does not secure. It attends to what is happening here and now—a very important task in everyday clinical medicine, to be sure—but has difficulty addressing underlying conditions that lead to problems in the first place. That is, by setting aside talk of (moral) theory and philosophy in lieu of "mid-level" principles, deep analysis of biomedical and moral conditions that underlie current situations is lost.

I would suggest the disconnected character of the principles from moral theory actually may arise from fact that there is no account of any philosophy or theory of medicine, as well. Why should that matter? Well, as Beauchamp and Childress themselves note, "we *draw from* the common morality to formulate these principles? To make them suitable *for biomedical ethics*" (2023, 151). In other words, the principles identified are not principles of the ethical life writ large, but of *biomedical* ethics, in particular. Even more directly, they purport to speak to the field of clinical medicine (and possibly other healthcare professions), as opposed to, say, research ethics which is covered by *The Belmont Report*. And yet, there is no place in their book where they take the time to explain what constitutes clinical medicine—what the aims, purposes, or scope of medicine itself are.

It is my contention that a look into what constitutes medicine and healthcare matters in light of a set of norms purporting to arise from and speak to biomedical practices. That is, a broader view looking into what medicine is about, in fact, may make principles of medicine more effective, and that work—the work of looking at the modern practice of medicine itself—was happening at the same time as the work of Beauchamp and Childress, but has been overshadowed—almost forgotten—by the normative work of principles.

I would hope it uncontroversial to say that the field of bioethics needed a *lingua franca*, a useful language available beyond the ethics experts. And yet, language is a fundamental characteristic of any culture (Dewey 1938). So, as a language develops, culture develops as well. During the 1970s, bioethics searched for its voice, with religionists, lawyers, philosophers, sociologists, and clinicians all contributing to the conversation. As we have noted, in the end, the language of principles, as articulated by two humanists, Tom Beauchamp (philosopher) and James Childress (religious ethicist), gave a framework in which that voice could express itself. But at the same time that the moral concerns that led Beauchamp and Childress to develop their model, others who recognized similar concerns took quite different tactics, and some of the leading voices who took dissimilar approaches were, themselves, physicians, not philosophers. Surprisingly, given that the profession in question is medicine, the approaches they took, while still influential among academic bioethicists, made little headway in how we think about clinical practice and clinical ethics for practicing clinicians who are outside the scholarly debates in bioethics.

Two such authors were Edmund Pellegrino and Eric Cassell, both practicing internists with rich backgrounds in philosophy and ethics, and both of whom began their work on the "nature" of medicine, clinical practice, and ethics in the decades preceding the '70s.

Edmund Pellegrino approached his philosophy of medicine and bioethics through an Aristotelian, virtue-based philosophy, reaching back to what he called Hippocratic values and filtered through a Catholic (more specifically, Thomasian) lens. An internist who began his work in the 1940s, Pellegrino was highly steeped in the humanities and always stayed within an academic environment, even becoming chancellor of Health Sciences at the University of Tennessee and president of the Catholic University of America, before ending his career at Georgetown seeing patients and doing bioethics at the Center for Clinical Bioethics at Georgetown, which is now named in his honor. Pellegrino's writings in medical and bioethics journals, along with his numerous books, place him squarely in the important moral conversations of a burgeoning field. He was a highly respected figure in the field of bioethics, earning recognition and honors throughout his career.

Much of the same can be said for Eric Cassell, whose career began in the 1950s, continuing until his death in 2021. Cassell was an internal medicine specialist and professor of public health at Weill Cornell Medical College. In 1971 he became a founding fellow at the Hastings Center, where he focused on issues at the end of life, laying groundwork for academic acceptance of palliative care. His book, *The Healer's Art* (1976), suggested that illness be seen by clinicians as transformative, not merely a problematic adjunct of living. And *The Nature of Suffering* (1991) became the seminal work on the topic of suffering, suggesting that it is a transformative experience to be taken seriously and individually by physicians.

With the great longevity of their careers, and their early infusion into academic bioethics, it is not unreasonable to think that, particularly *as physicians* themselves, either Pellegrino or Cassell, if not both, would have made a significant impact on how clinicians today understand the moral landscape of their practice. To be sure, writing important works during the nascent stage of professional bioethics, both Cassell and Pellegrino were significant parts of the academic discourse. And yet, by the end of the 1970s, two humanities professors set the course for moral evaluation of clinical practice in a way that nearly eliminated the effects of Cassell's and Pellegrino's insights, at least in terms of any impact of practicing clinicians.

Why might this be? I suggest that one powerful reason for this is that both Cassell and Pellegrino (in rather different ways) approach the ethical landscape of medicine, not through identifying moral norms of practice, but by discussing what they took to be the "nature" or "purpose" or "practice" of medicine itself. Again, this way of coming at the moral life of medicine is an approach somewhat ignored by Beauchamp and Childress. This contrast in approaches between Beauchamp and Childress, on the one hand, and Pellegrino and Cassell, on the other, is brought into stark relief if we take a brief moment to look at two chapter publications by Pellegrino and Cassell which came out in the same year as *The Principles*, 1979, in volume 6 of the book series, Philosophy and Medicine, entitled, *Clinical Judgment: A Critical Appraisal*.

The volume itself, edited by Engelhardt, Spicker, and Towers, is the result of a symposium on clinical judgment held in 1977. At the time, new pressures had arisen in medicine regarding the use of computers to aid in, even provide, diagnostics for clinicians (sound familiar in today's AI landscape?—for this reason alone, the volume is worth a close read even today). After two sections of debates discussing the role of diagnostic critical thinking and logic, computers, and human reasoning, the third section turns to insights on clinical judgment by clinicians themselves—namely, Pellegrino and Cassell.

What we learn, by implication if not always direct explication, through a careful reading of these chapters is that for both Pellegrino and Cassell clinical medicine is an inherently moral enterprise. Particularly in the case of Pellegrino, medicine is decidedly teleological, aimed (practically) at the "right healing action for a particular patient" (Pellegrino 1979, 173). As Karen Geraghty succinctly puts it, "[Pellegrino's] argument is deceptively simple: medicine is at heart a moral enterprise founded on the covenant of the patient-physician relationship" (2001). His account, then, of clinical judgment is necessarily infused with this "end," and as such, requires that the particularities of the patient themselves are necessary to identifying the "right healing action." As such, "[i]n making the 'right' decision for an individual patient..., personal, social, economic, and psychological characteristics of the patient must be factored in." (Pellegrino 1979, 181).

In his own chapter in the volume, Cassell focuses on the "subjective" considerations of patient themselves—note: not the subjective considerations of the physician, but the patient. Patients bring to the clinical encounter their experiences, beliefs, and feelings about their situation. Cassell suggests that clinicians, not in lieu of deep understanding of physiology and pathology but in order to use that understanding effectively, must "learn how the person of the patient interacts with basic pathologic mechanism to produce the illness that is *this* person with *this* disease" (205). Cassell argues that the subjective considerations of the patient must necessarily be a focus for the clinician because, "If [the physician] listens only to the sense data of the experiencer he [sic] will hear only about disease and will miss the person. If he hears only about the subjectivity he will miss the disease" (214).

In both Pellegrino's and Cassell's accounts, the argument for professional practice (habit) development requires a rich understanding of patients as both the everyday people they are and the patients they see themselves to be. Such a robust approach to the medical practice, which is the groundwork for the ethical landscape of medicine, is not to be found in the early editions of the *Principles*. Even as late as the fourth edition, Beauchamp and Childress suggest that respecting a patient is to focus on their autonomy through "express and informed consent" (1994, 128) which only lightly touches on the broader considerations of what it means for a clinician to respect the patient in front of them. Pellegrino and Cassell both call for a deeper understanding of the individual patient. To be fair, a moral concern for understanding who the patient is has not been wholly ignored; however, leaning into "then" rather than "thick" case descriptions (cf. Gavin 1995), much of the clinical ethics literature—especially articles and commentaries written for clinical journals, trades on principlist discussions of cases, not robust considerations of the "personal, social, economic, and psychological characteristics of the patient" as germane to moral medical practices.

To be clear, however, the point of my brief discussion of Cassell and Pellegrino and their views of medicine should not be taken as an endorsement of their specific philosophical accounts, per se, but instead is intended to suggest that a moral culture in medicine demands something more (not necessarily something other) than a principles-based approach to clinical ethics. An account of the moral life of medicine reduced to norms and precepts runs the risk of losing touch with the lived experiences of both patients and providers, becoming a "cookie cutter" approach to the conditions that manifest ethical concerns in medicine in the first place.

Taking my lead from pragmatist philosophy, phenomenology, and yes, people like Pellegrino and Cassell, back in the late 1990s I began arguing that the principle-based accounts of Beauchamp and Childress (and Engelhardt, for that matter) left us wanting because at least in their early incarnations, they mischaracterized the role of principles, the "nature" of autonomous humans. They ignored the importance of theory and philosophy for grounding an *ethical account of patient-provider relationships* in light of a pragmatic understanding of moral intelligence and artistry performed by socially situated selves which develop into and arises out of an attitude of community as healing. The following section, then, is a kind of precis of that argument.[2]

> Just in the degree in which a physician is an artist in his work he uses his science, no matter how extensive and accurate, to furnish him with tools of inquiry into the individual case, and with methods of forecasting a method of dealing with it. Just in the degree in which, no matter how great his learning, he subordinates the individual case to some classification of diseases and some generic rule of treatment, he sinks to the level of the routine mechanic. His intelligence and his action become rigid, dogmatic, instead of free and flexible. (MW12, 176)

As I've suggested, there is a need for an account of medicine as a profession, as a practice—a kind of philosophical expression of health care—and my work in bioethics starts from a philosophical grounding in American pragmatism. It is through this lens that I will argue for a more robust sense of medicine and ethics that acknowledges ethical norms but situates them within a more comprehensive context in which patient and providers reside in relationship to each other.

Pragmatism is a philosophical movement or "school" that arose in the late 19th and early 20th centuries. It included such figures as C. S. Peirce, William James, John Dewey, and George Mead (among others). While there is, of course, no one philosophical system that is "pragmatism," the "spirit" it captures can be found in a group of philosophical positions and theories that emphasize the practical outcomes of philosophical inquiry for human purposes. These outcomes and purposes arise from the intelligent and contextual nature of inquiry, take seriously the centrality and continuity of experience, and stress the evolution and habitual underpinnings of character. And though some may object to the fact that pragmatism is not clearly defined in one system, "The resistance of pragmatism to a precise definition is a mark of its vitality, an indication that it is a living philosophy rather than an historic relic" (Talisse and Aikin 2008, 3). Philosopher AO Lovejoy suggested over a century ago (1908) that there are at least "thirteen pragmatisms," but even so, most constructs of pragmatist philosophy aim at practical consequences, grounding in naturalism, recognition of fallibility, a belief in meliorism, and an integration of human thought and action. In light of these shared characteristics, many pragmatists

[2] The following section is a reduction/redaction from Hester (2001).

suggest that ideas, beliefs, and emotions are essentially biological and cultural habits. Habits trigger us to perform. Habits, defined as controlled adjustments between an individual and their environment, stand at the ready in order to manifest in specific situations. These acquired tendencies can be found in human action, thought, and emotion. For example, discovering a broken car window triggers a sequence of habitual reactions: blood rushing to the face, checking the watch, realizing missing electronics, and briskly walking back to the house while feeling frustrated and worried. These activities, driven by habits, are actions mobilized by circumstances. The violation of property activates habits of fear, frustration, investigation, and stress.

Habits are double-edged, though. While they make our efforts less taxing, their "automation" runs the risk of overwhelming reflection and intelligence. Let us call these thoughtless habits "habituations." They take the environment (at the time) as fixed and uniform; thus "adjustment is just fitting ourselves to this fixity of external conditions" (MW9, 51). Habituations are mechanical and routine.

> Habit as *habituation* is indeed something *relatively* passive.... Conformity to the environment, a change wrought in the organism without reference to ability to modify surroundings, is a marked trait of...habituations.... Habituation is...*our adjustment to an environment which at the time we are not concerned with modifying*. (MW9, 51–52 [emphasis added])

We can see this through how routine functions for practitioners[3] of medicine—from taking of vital signs to patient histories. Such habits are necessary for good medical care, but these and other habits become concerning if they are "set, rigid, and inflexible," leading to "unvarying behavior" (Columbia Associates in Philosophy 1923, 8). Such stagnation, what we might call 'habituations', can result in dogmatic physicians who "cannot successfully meet new situations" (Columbia Associates in Philosophy 1923, 8) precisely because patient differences need sensitive and adaptive responses. Dewey reminds us, "A habit marks an *inclination*—an active preference and choice for the conditions involved in its exercise." (MW9, 53) As "inclinations," habits "prefer" and "choose" the conditions that call them forth; they do not simply wait in reserve but seek out conditions in which to act. They attempt, at least upon first appearance, to be exercised in particular ways along very restricted lines. The active nature of habits can lead to the "unthinking" exercise of them. Again Dewey:

> Routine habits are unthinking habits.... [T]he acquiring of habits is due to an original plasticity of our natures: to our ability to vary responses till we find an appropriate and efficient way of acting. Routine habits, and habits that possess us instead of our possessing them, are habits which put an end to plasticity. They mark the close of power to vary. (MW9, 54)

However, let us not be fooled in to believing that habits undermine intelligence. In fact, habits and intelligence have an intimate, if paradoxical, relationship.

[3]Throughout I will use terms like 'medical practitioners', 'health care professionals', and 'physicians' interchangeably and do so to highlight that many of the issues discussed herein apply in varying degrees to MDs, DOs, APRNs, PAs, RNs, PTs, etc. alike.

> Habits are a condition of intellectual efficiency. They operate in two ways upon intellect. Obviously, they restrict its reach, they fix its boundaries.... All habit-forming involves the beginning of an intellectual speculation which if unchecked ends in thoughtless action....
>
> Habit is however more than a restriction of thought. Habits become negative limits because they are first positive agencies. The more numerous our habits the wider the field of possible observation and foretelling. The more flexible they are, the more refined is perception in its discrimination and the more delicate the presentation evoked by imagination. (MW14, 121 & 123)

Dewey contrasts habits unchecked by intelligence (for which they were initially placed into service) with flexible, productive habits that expand intellectual horizons. Let us call these productive habits "intelligent," serving as thoughtful and flexible manipulations nuanced in order to affect old habits in light of the uniqueness of each new situation.

> We are always possessed by habits and customs, and this fact signifies that we are always influenced by the inertia and the momentum of forces temporarily outgrown but nevertheless still present with us as a part of our being.... [However, i]n its largest sense,...remaking of the old through union with the new is precisely what intelligence is. (LW11, 36–37)

Given this, the medical profession, any more than other activities of life, cannot help but be replete with habits. And the tension between "unthinking" and "intelligent" habits also, then, exists in medicine. Unreflective approaches to patient care can run on virtually unchecked, from the expectations of physicians about their patients (and vice versa) to taking histories to using a stethoscope or palpating the abdomen, habits of medical practice make encounters with patients efficient but dangerous, possibly stifling positive, flexible interactions with unique individuals and situations.

Further, the institutions of medicine (from medical education to medical centers to medical insurance to ACOs) provide an environment in which habituations not only thrive but are even encouraged. At one time, HMOs used a term for time spent with patients—"medical-loss ratio," (Anders 1996), meaning that the medical encounter is to count as a negative loss from the standpoint of the "business" of medicine. Now days, RVUs (or RVWs) are the coin of the realm, with pressure on providers to "generate" high levels of RVUs—namely, patient encounters. But if institutions champion such metrics, then time is of the essence, where unthinking habits are more likely to run unchecked, since intelligent habits are typically more time-consuming than simple habituations.[4]

Now, equal to, if not more problematic than, turning the practitioner into a mechanical object, however, is the fact that the habituations of the practitioner must treat patients as categorizable problems, fitting into known groupings. The unique content of a patient's life-story—the "subjective," as Cassell puts it—is devalued, if not entirely lost. Without reflection in activity, medical personnel cannot account for the subtle but important differences among individual patients. In the life of everyday people, medicine often comes into play when someone is concerned about his/

[4] Sociologists Raymond DeVries and Peter Conrad have pointed out that bioethicsts themselves have paid far too little attention to the institutional environments in which medical practice becomes habituated and supported. See DeVries and Conrad (1998), (in particular) 235–237.

her health, and health is typically felt in intimate and sometimes even mortal/vital ways when in the midst of illness or injury. A cough may not simply mean a cold; it could spell pneumonia. A fast heartbeat could be the sign of over-exertion or critical heart problems. Patients come to doctors precisely because they sense these different possibilities even if they do not know them all. That is, each patient comes to medicine with their own unique experiences of the conditions they harbor.

Now, for some medical encounters, there certainly exist relatively "straightforward" occasions when neither party feels misunderstood or unsuccessful in reaching his/her goals. Stitching up a cut, dealing with a sinus infection, or setting a broken bone can, depending on the pervasive level of disruption in a patient's life, be instances where conditioned practice can work to all parties' satisfaction. And yet, there remains risk in even these "simple" cases, where the patient's own values, interests and pursuits (the surgeon with a broken finger, the singer with a sore throat) can turn the condition into something more than mere "routine" for them. And as cases get more complex—e.g., head injury, cancer, genetic disorders, congenital heart conditions, etc.—the chances of missing the boat both ethically and medically (if these two can be cleanly separated) increase if reflective care is not given.

Not simply bad personal interaction but *bad medicine* results from inattention to the differences and uniqueness of each case, each particular patient; in this both Pellegrino and Dewey agree. Each patient brings to the table a new situation never before encountered. Medicine, therefore, can never merely be a strict science of classification but an art-form that imaginatively applies the instruments of medical science based on careful investigation, dialectic, probability, and communication. Intelligent solutions require attention to the individual case, and clinical practice, in its attempt to bring about a healthy patient, is no less immune to the dangers of rote, dogmatic practice, than is any other occupation. "Medicine must not only perform well but act well, it must choose what should be done to heal a particular patient whose good is the true end of the whole activity" (Pellegrino 1979, 191). Science in its "pure" form relies on general principles and "scientific" medicine is no exception. But art is individual; it is unique. And medicine as an art-form must investigate and treat the individual patient, not a general type. "Medicine exists as medicine only when it engages in the *full range of activities* which constitute clinical judgment and which lead to decisive action in the interest of a *particular* patient" (Pellegrino 1979, 190 [emphasis added]). Dewy concurs,

> [Health] varies with [each person's] past experience, his opportunities, his temperamental and acquired weaknesses and abilities. Not man in general but a *particular* man suffering from some *particular* disability aims to live healthily, and consequently health cannot mean for him exactly what it means for any other mortal. Healthy living is not something to be attained by itself apart from other ways of living. A man needs to be healthy in his life, not apart from it, and what does life mean except the aggregate of his pursuits and activities? (1920, MW 12:175, emphasis added)

I argue, then, that medicine must develop a pragmatic understanding, or habits of intelligence, employed in the service of individual patients as they present themselves. In other words, medicine must rely on artistic methods which recognize the individuality of patients, an individuality which is developed out of the communities of which they are a part.

If this account is correct, then medicine must be seen necessarily as a moral enterprise because it is a practice focused on how people relate to each other, concerning the treatment of persons and the responsibility for that treatment. It is important, then, to inquire into not only the issue of habituation in practice but, further still, what kinds of habits and habituations should be developed and perpetuated in medicine in order to fashion moral encounters between medical professionals and patients. Rather than basing an account of moral rationality on principles and rules a richer account arises from an ethics based on imaginative, intelligent habits—what we might call "moral artistry."

In both medicine and ethics problem solving is often reduced to a formal process. Medically, we observe, gather information, apply norms and definitions, determine diagnoses and project outcomes. Ethical investigation, too, has been described as routine application of imperatives or principles, the following of rules and order. But such descriptions belie the fact that much imaginative activity is involved. Of course, truly *rigid* routine has little place in intelligent activity. As such both medical and moral deliberation, itself, cannot be rote application of principles and rules, it must be creatively flexible and adaptive. For Dewey, ethics concerns all aspects of moral living—values (character), duties (roles), and goods (ends). We might say, then, the "field" of ethics—i.e., the territory of values and interests covered by moral considerations—comprises those *evaluations* of human (and some other animal) conduct, both arising from and affecting character, which result in appraisals of "good" and "bad," "right" and "wrong." Moral considerations must take ends seriously, but those ends are inextricably tied to motivations and means, character and action. Thus, both what constitutes a "good" and what constitutes appropriate ways to achieve our goods are open for debate because "it is the characteristic of any situation properly called moral that one is ignorant of the end and of good consequences, of the right and just approach, of the direction of virtuous conduct, and that one must search for them" (1930, LW5 280)

In the face of this challenge of the moral life, a pragmatic account of deliberation begins with

> our capacity for *imagination.* Imagination, like *drama,* is story-structured and is spurred by conflicts and contrasts among characters and contingent events.... Rather than being a lyric outburst, imagination (and thus the aesthetic) is constrained and guided by the exigencies and pressures of a situation along with our vast array of internalized *social habits.* (Fesmire 1995, 569–570)

As Dewey himself says, "deliberation is a dramatic rehearsal (in imagination) of various compelling possible lines of action" (MW14, 132).

The imagination, then, has a moral function since "[i]n language and imagination *we rehearse the response of others* just as we dramatically enact other consequences." (MW14, 216 [emphasis added]) This "story-structured" capacity "guided by" environmental pressures, cultural institutions, and social habits helps us deliberate among a variety of ends-in-view in order to choose a particular path to follow. "For deliberation to be brought to a dramatic resolution, it must develop so as to have a form that expresses coherently the conflicts that originally set the problem of inquiry." (Fesmire 1995, 570). Moral deliberation, thus, starts from particular problems in order to develop a coherent story. Specifically, particular problems are characterized by conflict with existent conditions. Moral deliberation through imagination works, in part, to develop a coherent story (or "narrative") that adequately "expresses" the conflicts which characterize the particular problem to be solved. And here, it might be best to understand, for moral purposes, the term "coherence" in a particular way.

On this traditional account of morality, there is an attempt to create one universal rational scheme—be it deontology or utilitarian or other—where "right" and "good" are defined rationally or "by nature" in a way that our deliberations must comport with these a priori notions. Pragmatists, however, start with a framework where "right" and "good" are the results of the end of inquiry and moral deliberation, not the beginnings, and as such, will only arise after careful consideration of all persons affected by the current situation and the consequences of our proposed actions. In this light, deliberation must attempt to *create* a narrative that includes as many concrete interests as possible. Philosopher William James states succinctly, "*Invent some manner* of realizing your own ideals which will also satisfy the alien demands—that and only that is the path to peace" (James [1897], 623). In other words, the narrative of the moral situation should include disparate but relevant narratives in its account. Steve Fesmire suggests that this be done by setting ourselves in the place of the other:

> [A]..."complete" dramatic rehearsal strives to weave the interests and purposes of ourselves and others into an integrated and enduring tapestry. Hence, not only must we forecast consequences for ourselves, but also, ... we must (and do) dramatically play the role of others whose lives interlace with our own. We must imaginatively project ourselves into the emerging dramas of *their* lives to discover how their life-stories or 'narrative' may be meaningfully continued alongside our own. Immoral conduct is thus not merely a deficiency in one's capacity to follow moral laws or rules. Much more than this, immorality stems from a scarcity of moral imagination and a failure in moral artistry. (Fesmire 1995, 571)

Dramatic rehearsal in imagination, then, leads to moral artistry through the weaving of coherent narratives that take the other in his/her desires seriously. As such, m*oral activity is not easy*. Fortunately, however, moral artistry can be understood as the imaginative use of habits of intelligence in everyday social situations. The moral artist never merely attempts to apply abstract rules or principles; s/he learns to view problems through habits of intelligence that creatively and dramatically rehearse possible solutions to problematic situations at hand, adjusting desires and the situation in order to develop a story that takes the other seriously. "Deliberation is not a mathematical utilitarian calculation, nor is it a Kantian determinate judgment; it has a dramatic *story to tell.*" (Fesmire 1995, 574 [emphasis added])

> Stanley Hauerwas and David Burrell expand this even further, for like Dewey, they say,
>
> There can be no [one] normative theory of the moral life that is sufficient to capture the rich texture of the many moral notions we inherit. What we actually possess are various and

> sometimes conflicting stories that provide us with the many skills to use certain moral notions. What we need to develop is the reflective capacity to analyze those stories, so that we better understand how they function. (Burrell and Hauerwas 1989, 170)

Hauerwas and Burrell note that morality is not simply about isolated individuals and their desires and stories, but in order to develop moral rationality, we must pay close attention to stories.

With such an account of morality's connection with narrative, important implications follow for medical encounters. As important as any insight we might have is this: Bioethical theories like that of Beauchamp and Childress have been based primarily on Enlightenment conceptions of the self, treating selves as insular and atomic. In such a scheme individual patients are empowered primarily through the act of "free and informed" consent, leaving the patient in a passive state. *However*, narrative accounts of morality challenge this account of the self, arguing instead that the self is insulated, but is itself a product of social interaction, evolving and adjusting as the story moves through its context. *The self is not an unchanging entity* at the core of each human being *but is a process and function*—let's call it a "narrative"—which develops and changes as individuals learn to adapt to and manipulate the world around them.

As Larry Churchill notes, "Narrative is a profound mode for understanding … because it forces us to attend to the human voices, including our own, behind what is being said" (2014). Seeing people (in particular, patients) as narratives affects our moral approach to patient care. Dewey tells us,

> [T]he discovery that a man [sic.] is suffering from an illness is not a discovery that he must suffer, or that the subsequent course of events is determined by his illness; it is the indication of a needed and a possible course by which to restore health. Even the discovery that the illness is hopeless falls within this principle. It is an indication not to waste time and money on certain fruitless endeavors, to prepare affairs with respect to death, etc. It is also an indication to search for conditions which will render in the future similar cases remediable, not hopeless. The whole case…stands or falls with this principle [namely, that facts are contextual and call for an intelligently determined response]. (MW 8, 18–19)

As such, the role of narrative in the medical and moral consideration of the patient is that "Narratives represent events not as general laws but rather as elements of a history where a continuing individual or collective subject suffers or brings about dramatic, i.e. meaningful, changes. A change is meaningful in relation to past *and future events*" (Bernstein 1990). Clinicians must, then, approach medicine with imaginative moral artistry of creatively intelligent persons. This is an active process of involvement in the current circumstances and future pursuits expressed and required in the situation at hand. Thereby, the engaged participant, and not the passive, consenting patient, becomes our "model" for clinicians and patients alike. Together, healthcare professionals and patients pursue desired ends that, as Pellegrino states it, are the right healing actions for particular patients, and as Cassell points out, treats the patient for the subject, not object.

Something got lost along the way in the development of contemporary bioethics. The loss, I would suggest, is profound. It has affected the education of medical trainees since the 1980s. While bioethics certainly needed to find its disciplinary footing, its acceptance and reification of basic principles (while necessary) had the effect of reducing, if not eliminating, a richer account of the moral space of medicine. The insights of writers like Pellegrino and Cassell (among others, to be sure) are practically missing for generations of clinicians. And yet what they pointed to as clinicians themselves was the need for a broad account of the moral considerations within medical encounters, an account that can include and yet goes beyond basic norms and precepts to an expectation of a robust consideration of the full character of the people and conditions that make-up the encounter itself. This, I have argued, acknowledges that patients are not insular beings but contextually narrative beings, and thus our moral approach to medicine requires a moral imagination and artistry that aims to help individuals live healthily within the unique and collective contexts through which they become the individuals they are.

References[5]

Anders, George. 1996. *Health Against Wealth: HMOs and the Breakdown of Medical Trust*. Houghton Mifflin.

Baker, R. 2024. *Making Modern Medical Ethics: How African Americans, Anti-Nazis, Bureaucrats, Feminists, Veterans, and Whistleblowing Moralists Created Bioethics*. The MIT Press.

Beauchamp, T., and J. Childress. 1979. *Principles of Biomedical Ethics*. 1st ed. Oxford University Press. 4th ed. 1994.

Bernstein, J. M. 1990. Self-knowledge as Praxis: Narrative and Narration in Psychoanalysis. In *Narrative in Culture*, ed. C. Nash. Routledge.

Burrell, D., and S. Hauerwas. 1989. From System to Story: An Alternative Pattern for Rationality in Ethics. In *Why Narrative? Readings in Narrative Theology*, ed. S. Hauwerwas and L. G. Jones, 158–190. W. B. Eerdmans.

Cassell, E. J. 1976. *The Healer's Art*. The MIT Press.

Cassell, E. J. 1979. The Subjective in Clinical Judgment. In *Clinical Judgment: A Critical Appraisal*, ed. H. T. Engelhardt et al., 199–215. D. Reidel Publishing.

Churchill, L. 2014. Narrative Awareness in Ethics Consultations: The Ethics Consultant as Story-Maker. *Hasting Center Report* 44 (Suppl. 1): S36–S39.

Columbia Associates in Philosophy. 1923. *Introduction to Reflective Thinking*. Houghton Mifflin Co.

DeVries, R., and P. Conrad. 1998. Why Bioethics Needs Sociology. In *Bioethics and Society*, ed. R. DeVries and J. Subedi, 233–257.

Dewey, John. 1915. *The Logic of Judgments in Practice*. MW 8.

Dewey, John. 1916. *Democracy and Education*. MW 9.

[5] Citations of John Dewey's works are to the thirty-seven-volume critical edition published by Southern Illinois University Press under the editorship of Jo Ann Boydston. In-text citations give the original publication date, series abbreviation, followed by volume number and page number. For example: (1934, LW 10:12) is page 12 of *Art as Experience*, which is published as volume 10 of *The Later Works*.

Series abbreviations for *The Collected Works*.

EW *The Early Works* (1882–98).

MW *The Middle Works* (1899–1924).

LW *The Later Works* (1925–53).

Dewey, John. 1922. *Human Nature and Conduct*. MW 14.
Dewey, John. 1930. *Three Independent Factors in Morals*. LW 5.
Dewey, John. 1935. *Liberalism and Social Action*. LW 11.
Dewey, John. 1938. *Logic: A Theory of Inquiry*. LW 12.
Evans, J. H. 2012. *The History and Future of Bioethics: A Sociological View*. Oxford University Press.
Fesmire, S. 1995. Dramatic Rehearsal and the Moral Artist: A Deweyan Theory of Moral Understanding. *Transactions of the Charles S. Peirce Society* 21:568–597.
Fletcher, Joseph. 1954. *Morals and Medicine*. Boston: Beacon Press.
Gavin, W. J. 1995. *Cuttin' the Body Loose*. Temple University Press.
Geraghty, K. 2001. Commemorative Issues: Guarding the Art, Edmund D Pellegrino, MD. *AMA: Virtual Mentor* 3:405–407.
Hester, D. M. 2001. *Community as Healing: Pragmatist Ethics in Medical Encounters*. Rowman & Littlefield.
James, W. 1897. The Moral Philospher and the Moral Life. *The Will to Believe and Other Essays in Popular Philosophy*, Longmans, Green, and Co., 184–215.
Jonsen, A. 1997. The Birth of Bioethics: The Origins and Evolution of a Demi-discipline. *Medical Humanities Review* 11 (1): 9–21.
Lovejoy, A. O. 1908. The Thirteen Pragmatisms. In *The Thirteen Pragmatisms: and Other Essays*, ed. A. O. Lovejoy. The Johns Hopkins Press.
Pellegrino, E. D. 1979. Anatomy of a Clinical Judgment: Some Notes on Right Reason and Right Action. In *Clinical Judgment: A Critical Appraisal*, ed. H. T. Engelhardt Jr. et al., 169–194. D. Reidel Publishing.
Talisse, Robert B., and Scott F. Aikin. 2008. *Pragmatism: A Guide for the Perplexed*. London: Continuum.

Chapter 11
The Anatomy of Clinical Judgments: Some Notes on Right Reason and Right Action

Edmund D. Pellegrino

For it is uneducated not to have an eye for when it is necessary to look for proof and when this is not necessary.

Aristotle (1940, Metaphysics IV, 1006a)

11.1 Introduction

Richard Cabot, one of the most celebrated of American diagnosticians, labelled his attempts to anatomize the process of differential diagnosis "a very dangerous topic – dangerous to the reputation of physicians for wisdom…. Physicians are naturally reluctant on such matters, slow to put their thoughts to paper, and very suspicious of any attempts to tabulate their methods of reasoning" (Cabot 1916, 19).

Sixty years later most clinicians remain reluctant and more than a little suspicious. Many still take refuge in the "art" and its exclusive mysteries, to resist formalization of their mental operations. In recent years, the "dangerous" subject has been boldly attacked by a few clinicians with unusual facility in the language of

This chapter originally appeared as Edmund D. Pellegrino, "The Anatomy of Clinical Judgments. Some Notes On Right Reason And Right Action," in *Clinical Judgment: A Critical Appraisal*, ed. H.T. Engelhardt, Jr., et al. (D. Reidel Publishing, 169–194. Reprinted with permission from Springer.

Edmund D. Pellegrino died before publication of this work was completed.

E. D. Pellegrino (✉)
New Haven, CT, USA

L. M. Rasmussen, S. Holm (eds.), *50 Years of Philosophy and Medicine*,
Philosophy and Medicine 150, https://doi.org/10.1007/978-3-031-95175-6_11

logic and statistics so that dissection of the tangle of science, art and conjecture is now well underway (Black 1968, 17–19; Feinstein forthcoming; Jacquez 1964; Ledley and Lusted 1959; Murphy 1976; Wulff 1976). They have been joined by statisticians, engineers, psychologists, and philosophers who are bringing the more sophisticated techniques of their disciplines to bear on this important and complex question.

Physicians and philosophers have puzzled for a long time over the nature of the physician's enterprise. Its dissection began with the Hippocratic physicians who first insisted on the primacy of observations of patients, refined by reason. They thus made medicine a natural science, separating it from both philosophy and religion with which it had so long been intimately associated (Jaeger 1944, 17-19).

Intuitive, hieratic, artistic and even magical elements of the physician's enterprise were not so easily removed however. Celsus, the Roman Hippocrates, spoke of medicine as an "ars coniecturalis"; William Osler, the modern Hippocrates, deemed it "… a science of uncertainty and an art of probability." Medicine has yet to become a science comparable in method and explanatory power with the laboratory sciences – though this is the expressed aim of some of our contemporary thinkers.

The puzzlement continues today in the growing tension between the scientific-actuarial and the artist-intuitionist models of clinical judgment (Elstein 1976). Each view tries earnestly to understand, and thus to improve, the clinical enterprise. One seeks to transform the conjectural elements into respectable science by formal analysis in terms of probabilistic logic or decision theory. Meanwhile, the other declares the nuances of clinical judgment to be an art, insusceptible to formal analysis, and improvable only by cultivation as one cultivates painting, music or sculpture.

This essay undertakes nothing so pretentious as the resolution of what seems to be a polemically seductive polarity in viewpoints. It takes the view that: Clinical decisions can be made more rigorous logically, without reducing everything to algorithm and regression equations. While much of the process remains opaque and insusceptible to extant methods of formal analysis, this need not forever be the case.

Much of the polarization between explanations of clinical judgment seems avoidable, if two significant features which have been neglected are sufficiently taken into account. These are: First, the over-riding fact that the whole process is ordained to a specific practical end – a right action for a particular patient – and that this end must modulate each step leading to it in important ways. A value screen is thus, in a way, cast over the entire sequence. Second is the fact that no unitary explanation or logical method can encompass the several different reasoning modes and several kinds of evidence acceptable in answering the different kinds of questions the clinician must answer.

The aim of this paper is *not* to countermand the utility of scientific actuarial formulations, or offer in their stead a benignant eclecticism which allows equal place to the explicable and inexplicable, i.e., to the "science" and the "art" of clinical judgment. Rather, it hopes to locate more precisely the several reasoning modes useful at each of the sequential and simultaneous steps which eventuate ultimately in a clinical action. This localization constitutes the anatomy of clinical judgment, an essential foundation for further formalization of the process.

The complete process is a multi-step, end-oriented concatenation of decisions demanding different types of reasons and reasonings which will justify a particular course of action, for a particular patient, given that patient's particular existential situation at the time of the decision. Each step is shot through with uncertainties, some eradicable, some not. Selection of the "right" action requires optimization of these uncertainty states.

Inasmuch as the nature of the uncertainties varies, the logical instruments used to achieve optimization will vary also. Thus, the methods of deductive and inductive reasoning, of dialectic, ethics and rhetoric are each appropriate to some step. Prudent and judicious action, rather than a true statement or scientific law, is the end to which the whole is directed. No one kind of evidence is universally applicable, and no single logical or epistemic mode suffices for all.

Customarily, discussion of clinical judgment ends at the establishment of the most probable diagnosis, or at best at the selection of a treatment. The third step – whether the treatment selected ought to be instituted, how, when, under what conditions – is usually not formally analyzed. Yet, one cannot speak legitimately of clinical judgment without seeing the whole process, particularly the way the end conditions the steps that precede it.

Four questions must be examined to sustain these assertions:

(1) What is the character of the end of clinical judgment?
(2) What questions must be answered in attaining that end?
(3) How does the end project itself on each step, i.e., what kinds of reasons does it require?
(4) What are the theoretical and practical implications of the proposed view of clinical judgment?

The answers bear to some extent on the difficult problem of a general theory of medicine. Such a theory must account for the full range of medical activity – seeking general laws of disease and treatment, but also taking specific actions in the interest of specific patients. Science, art, and the virtue of prudence infuse the several operations. But medicine justifies itself uniquely as medicine – as opposed to medicine as clinical or basic science, or as the art of performing medical acts – when it ends in a decision to act for, and in behalf of, a human who seeks to be healed (Pellegrino 1976a, b). To the extent that it identifies features which distinguish medicine from other human activities, the analysis of clinical judgment can contribute to the emerging structure of a theory of medicine.

11.2 What Is the End of Clinical Reasoning?

When a patient consults a physician, he/she does so with one specific purpose in mind: to be healed, to be restored and made whole, i.e., to be relieved of some noxious element in his/her physical or emotional life which the patient defines as disease – a distortion of his/her accustomed perception of what is a satisfactory life.

Usually some event has occurred – pain, lack of appetite, fatigue, trauma, a lump, spitting blood – some sign or symptom which exceeds a certain highly personalized threshold of tolerance in such fashion as to compromise, obstruct or discolor the person's perception of him/herself and his/her health. At the point when this perception leads to the *need* to be healed, the person becomes a *patient.* This transition has two existential connotations crucial to this discussion. Becoming a patient is to become one who suffers (patior, pati), and simultaneously one to whom something is done, a recipient as distinguished from an agent (O.E.D.). The patient, then, is a suffering person who comes to the physician to have something done to assist him/her to regain his/her former state or a more optimal one.

It is important to interject here that the term "patient" does not necessarily imply a passive restoration in which the physician is the sole agent. The patient ideally also participates in the restoration. He/she is seen as bearing a burden of illness which requires some action or decision mutually arrived at for cure to take place. The patient can yield his/her moral agency to the physician only by direct mandate. Only in the rarest circumstances will the physician legitimately be the patient's moral agent (MacIntyre 1977; Pellegrino 1977).

The end of the medical encounter, and the process of clinical judgment through which it is achieved then, is restoration and healing – some corrective, remedial or preventive action is directed at what the doctor and the patient perceive as a diminution of the patient's wholeness, each in his/her own fashion. The end is not a diagnosis, a scientific truth, testing an hypothesis or evaluating a treatment, though the knowledge derived therefrom enters into several states in making the decision to act.

The clinical decision comes at the end of a chain of deductive and inductive inferences, serially modified by recourse to "facts" and observations, usually themselves to some degree uncertain. Truth and certitude are, therefore, almost always problematic. Out of the uncertain conclusions of earlier syllogisms, a decision to act must be taken which has a different character from the conclusions that precede it. The conclusions of the earlier reasoning chains become premises for further reasoning. This is the normal condition of scientific reasoning – a cumulative and progressive series of hypotheses and conclusions, always open to further recourse to fact and experiment.

Each clinical decision is, however, a terminal and unique event in that it cannot remain forever open and it is not universalizable. It must close on the selection of one or a series of remedial actions – or none. The action chosen must be the "*right*" one for this patient. That is to say, it must be as congruent as possible with his/her particular clinical context, his/her values and his/her sense of what is "worthwhile" or "good". What the physician and the patient seek together is a judicious decision, one which optimizes as many benefits and minimizes as many risks as the situation will allow. The definition of risk is highly personal, and it turns on the patient's estimate of a danger "worth" running. The end is, therefore, not a general statement of the probabilities, but a particular statement of what a particular patient *should* do.

The criteria of a right or good decision lie not in its certitude, rigor, logical or mathematical soundness, though the probability of a judicious action is enhanced greatly when these qualities in here in the prior conclusions on which it is built.

These qualities must be secured wherever possible, but they are not sufficient for a "right" decision. They can, on the view I am propounding, be displaced or modulated by the more complex criteria of a decision "good" for this patient – what among the many things that *can* be done *ought* to be done?

Clearly, value considerations and moral issues – for both the patient and the physician – can color the selection of the facts and reasons which justify placing one diagnosis over another, the justifications accepted for taking action, and the degree to which the physician persuades or the patient assents to the final decision. The end must therefore be understood in all its fullness, because it projects itself so forcefully on the entire sequence.

The primary end of clinical judgment – a right healing action for a particular patient – imposes an atmosphere of prudence, over the whole process. Truth, for the practical intellect, is rightness with respect to human deeds, those dependent upon human will and intention. It differs thus from the truth of science which is a certain conformity with the reality it seeks to explain, and art, with the product it wishes to produce.

It is the end of medical judgment which also gives authenticity to the professions a physician makes – that he/she will use his/her knowledge and skill to "heal", according to the fullness of meaning of the word for his/her patient. Not to keep that end paramount is to make an inauthentic – indeed an immoral – profession. Medicine qua medicine is then more than a clinical or basic science applied to individual cases. It is a particularized knowledge of prudent healing actions, dependent upon scientific methods and art, but not synonymous with them.

Whatever formal analysis one favors – traditional syllogistics, the logic of probabilities, Bayesian conditional probabilities, decision analysis theory, information processing models, or judicial algorithms – each must account for the modulation and shaping imposed by the end. This would be so even if a high degree of certitude were possible at every step. Usually, however, we deal with varying "degrees of belief," and the judicious choice of actions becomes an even more critical and sensitive activity, difficult to formalize and formularize.

11.3 What Questions Must Be Addressed and with What Reasoning Modes?

When a person becomes a patient in the sense we have defined that state, a whole series of questions becomes crucial for him/her as a knowing and valuing being. What is wrong? Is it serious? What will it mean to me? Can it be cured, and by what means? Is the cure worthwhile? What will it cost? What *should* I do? These and corollary questions must be addressed if the process of clinical judgment is to be a complete and authentic medical judgment. They are reducible to three *generic* questions: *What can be wrong? What can be done? What should be done for this patient?* (Fig. 11.1) Let us look briefly at each question to see the kinds of reasoning relevant to each question, and what kinds of justifications are acceptable.

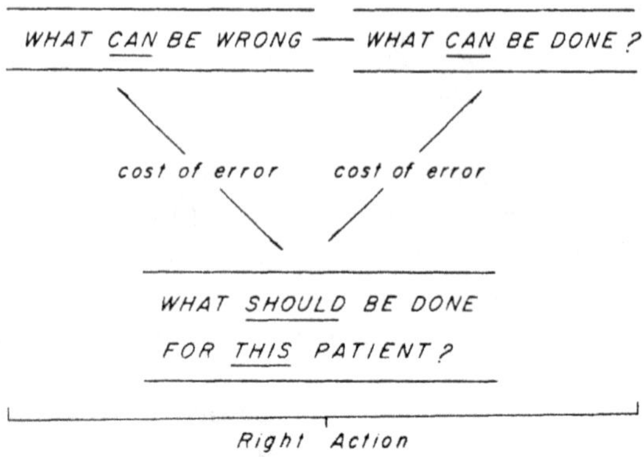

Fig. 11.1 What can be wrong? What can be done? What should be done for this patient?

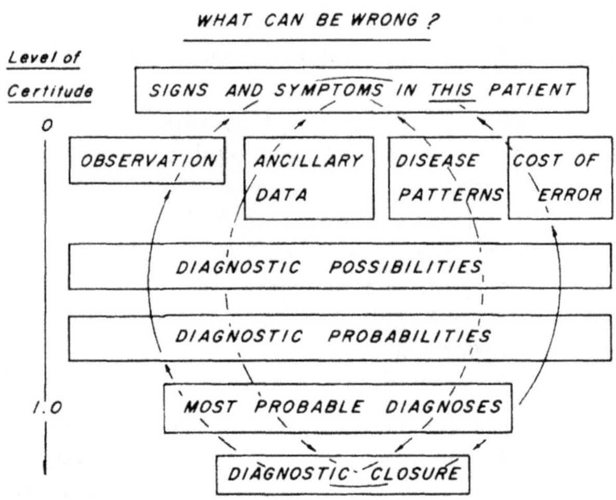

Fig. 11.2 What can be wrong?

11.3.1 What Can Be Wrong? (Fig. 11.2)

This is the diagnostic and classificatory question – the first part of the process and the one which has received the most vigorous theoretical examination. Given the signs and symptoms presented by this patient, what classificatory patterns fit best? Of the possible patterns, which is most probable, and with what degree of certainty?

This part of the process most closely fits the scientific paradigm and under ideal conditions can yield a diagnostic conclusion with a high degree of certitude – i.e., the error rate approaches zero. The conditions for such certitude must be stringent, however. The input data of signs and symptoms must be reliably observed, standardized and specified; the classificatory patterns must be equally reliably determined; the probabilities of different combinations of signs and symptoms must be derived from sufficient numbers and combinations of sets and subsets of signs and symptoms; laboratory and other ancillary data must be sensitive, accurate, specific and precise. The rules of deductive or probabilistic logic must be followed rigorously.

In addition, a highly specific and sharply discriminating test is required – like a biopsy, fiber endoscopy, angiography, or an enzymatic or immunological determination. Where all these conditions are met, *diagnostic closure* can be obtained. This means that all essential criteria for a diagnosis have been met. The diagnosis could even meet the test of scientific "elegance" if it is arrived at with an economy of steps.

These rigorous conditions are only rarely satisfied in clinical reality. Bedside data are notoriously unstandardized and poorly quantified (Koran 1975a, b); laboratory tests very widely in sensitivity, specificity, reliability and accuracy (McNeil et al. 1975); "Almost all data on the general incidence and prevalence of disease are inaccurate" (Feinstein 1967, 214). Even less secure are estimates of the cost of error of a clinical act so that the hopes of decision theorists to assign a numerical value to every nodal point in a decision tree are even less secure (Sokal 1964; Raiffa 1968; Feinstein forthcoming). Finally, probability statements say something about the population of individuals sharing some common characteristic but they are weakest in their description of the actual state of any individual in that population.

Thus, even when the rules of probabilistic logic are rigorously applied the diagnostic conclusions are still open to question. They are, more often than not, tentative "working" diagnoses and have more the quality of opinions than scientific judgments (Weaver 1968, 101–117). Adding more empiric data may as easily compound an error as move the conclusion closer to the asymptote of a true statement. At some point adding more tests adds only marginally to certitude if at all.

Differential diagnosis consists then in the selection of some diagnosis as more probable, or more justifying of an action than others. At some point, every diagnosis must proceed without further recourse to empirical input. The strength of the case for each diagnostic claim must be assessable and put in some order of priority against the others. Why, for example, is this chest pain due to angina pectoris and not to the fifty or more other kinds of chest pain? The selection must be made when all the empiric data are "in", and further appeals to the empiric are either impossible or insufficient to bring us any closer to diagnostic closure. This part of the differential diagnostic process is not synonymous with application of the laws of statistical probability. Indeed, a critique of the statistical argument as one among other arguments is itself requisite.

The process of differential diagnosis is really most akin to the process of classical dialectic (Adler 1927, 31, footnote 1 and 243–247). Each diagnostic possibility can be seen as a "claim"; the strength of arguments for, and against, each claim is evaluated; each position is clarified and set against its opposite; the inherent logical probity of each is delineated. Dialectical discourse properly conducted becomes an internal soliloquy in which the clinician examines his own conclusions critically, or tests them externally against his colleagues or consultants. No new truths are discovered this way, and the dialectic ends if an appeal to experience is possible. The process is therefore not "scientific" in either the classical or modern sense of science.

Differential diagnosis is usually addressed as synonymous with an assessment of relative probabilities. Yet part of the dialectical procedure is to examine the probity of the statistical method itself. When the facts are not determinative, we must establish which diagnostic claim has the strongest logical position. This is more akin to arguing a case in court than it is to proving a scientific hypothesis. The whole effort is to make one diagnosis sufficiently more cogent than the others so that it becomes a defensible basis for decisive action.

The dialectical process is especially important in science where it has been shown that psychologically the tendency is to prove rather than disprove one hypothesis (Sober 1978). New possibilities are often uncovered only by disproving an existing hypothesis entirely. Dialectical discourse assures an adversarial stance which challenges the tendency to settle too easily for a merely "workable" hypothesis.

The "old-fashioned" clinico-pathological conference was primarily an exercise in clinical dialectic. It has fallen into disrepute, yet it remains an invaluable way to teach the process of internal soliloquizing which enables the diagnostician to examine his own reasoning critically, when the possibility of adding more observations and tests is no longer open to him. Contemporary pedagogical opinion to the contrary, the dialectical discourse of a clinico-pathological exercise more closely approximates the clinical conditions of differential diagnosis than the scientific model of serial hypothesis testing.

In answering the first of the triad of questions that make up a clinical judgment, several different kinds of reasoning, and reasons, must be employed. To understand the pathophysiology of clinical manifestations, to define and apply a classificatory schema, "scientific" reasons are appropriate. To make general statements of probability for populations, statistical logic is needed. In differential diagnosis the rules of dialectic are the most pertinent. Uncertainty pervades every step of the diagnostic process from its epistemological assumptions to its logical operations. Each of several reasoning modes is suited to optimizing different forms of uncertainty. In the next section we shall see how the practical end modifies each of these modes at every step.

11.3.2 What Can Be Done? (Fig. 11.3)

This is the therapeutic question. Having made some decision about the nature of the patient's problem, what kinds of actions could be taken to remove or ameliorate the probable disorder?

Here again, the process is in part, and under certain stringent conditions, scientific in character. When there is a verifiable data base on the course of the untreated disease, and its modification by drugs, surgery, diet or other measure, the conditions for a scientific decision can be fulfilled. Equally indispensable are quantifiable and precise information about effectiveness and toxicity, since these must be weighed against each other before the decision is made. Under these conditions "closure" on a therapeutic action can approach certitude.

The therapeutic decision is easy to make when there is a specific and highly effective treatment which demonstrably alters the natural history of the disease. Penicillin for pneumococcal pneumonia, isoniazide and PAS for tuberculous

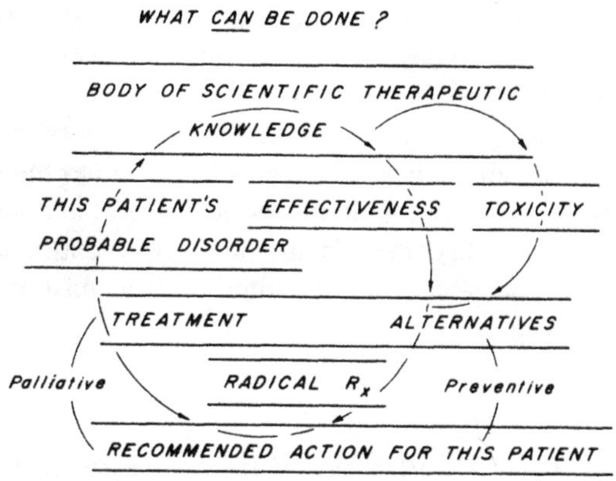

Fig. 11.3 What can be done?

meningitis, vitamin B12 for pernicious anemia, or abdominal surgery for ruptured peptic ulcer are examples. In these instances, the action recommended can be scientifically validated, and it will in most instances take precedence over other considerations. The recommended procedure then becomes synonymous with right action, and little choice is open to patient or physician, though the patient may in extreme circumstances reject even this kind of advice.

Unfortunately, to a much larger degree than in diagnostic decisions, genuinely scientific information in therapeutics is scanty. The many pitfalls of therapeutic trials have been the subject of a vast literature. They are generally acknowledged to be among the most difficult experiments to design, control, carry out and interpret. Even the randomized clinical trial has come under fire recently (Feinstein and Wells forthcoming). Especially problematic are the large number of therapeutic maneuvers which are not *radical* – i.e., they do not eradicate the causal agent or the offending process. Their benefits, if any, are marginal and the ratio of risk to benefit often vacillates widely. One has only to recall the sad history of anticoagulants in myocardial infarction, the recent national dilemma about influenza vaccination, or the belated appreciation of the long-term vascular effects of oral contraceptives or antidiabetic agents.

Today, we must often decide whether to recommend complex, expensive, palliative procedures with unpleasant and dangerous side effects – as in chemotherapy for cancer. Data on effectiveness and toxicity are usually available in these circumstances, but the questions are a different order: Is the discomfort worthwhile for this patient? Is length of life more important to him or her than its quality? This kind of question must rest firmly on scientific data, but that is only the foundation for a discussion permeated by the physician's and the patient's value systems.

The therapeutic and prognostic domains may well be, as Feinstein opines, the truly unique elements of clinical science. They are also the least secure scientifically. We simply lack the long-term observations of carefully selected patients in sufficient numbers to warrant secure prognostications about the course of a particular disease in a particular patient. Without such data, it is impossible to ground effectiveness of any agent scientifically unless it is so radically effective that a few cases will suffice. If the untreated mortality is 100%, any change will indicate effectiveness, as it does in treating subacute bacterial endocarditis or tuberculous meningitis with specific antibiotics.

The choice of what action to recommend involves more questions of value, by far, than diagnosis. The closer we come to the end of the process of clinical judgment – the right action – the less useful and less available is the scientific model. Reasoning becomes, in smaller part, scientific and probabilistic, and in larger part, dialectical – arguing one alternative against another without recourse to new factual data.

11.3.3 What Should Be Done for This Patient? (Fig. 11.4)

Having decided what the probable diagnosis is, and what treatment can be expected to be most effective and least harmful, the final question in clinical judgment is whether the treatment *should* be used in this patient, and what alternatives can be offered. The right action – the best one for a given patient – is not always synonymous with the logically or scientifically deduced action. The amount and kind of information needed to secure a diagnosis may be quite different from that needed for decisive action. It is the task of the last stage of clinical judgment to make these distinctions with as much precision as possible.

Decisive action frequently involves the counter position of what is good scientifically, what the physician *thinks* is good, and what the patient will accept as good. Scientific, personal and professional values intersect each other and can be in conflict. The scientific evidence and the probability statements about diagnosis,

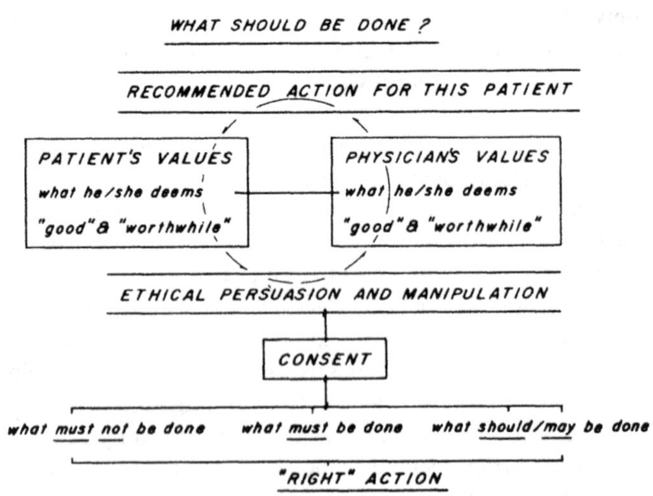

Fig. 11.4 What should be done for this patient?

prognosis and treatment become arguments for or against a choice of alternatives – to do nothing, or, if something is to be done, what must be done, what may be done, and what should be done.

If the patient exhibits the minimal criteria for an acute abdomen, signs of intracranial pressure, a stab wound of the heart, he/she *must* be operated upon; with severe blood loss, bacterial endocarditis, tuberculous meningitis, or diabetic coma proper, medical therapy *must* be instituted. On the other hand, a non-strangulated hernia, symptomatic gall stones, or mildly symptomatic benign prostatic hypertrophy are things that *should be* treated but may not be in the *must* category. Finally, hemorrhoids, varicose veins or lipomata *may be* removed surgically; or mild hypertension, a cold or sinusitis *may be* treated, but need not be.

When it comes to making the *right* decision – the *judicious* one for this patient – the categories of *must not, must, should* and *may* can all shift, depending upon a myriad of factors in the patient's life situation and his/her notion of what he/she deems worthwhile. In the more obvious situation – like a Jehovah's Witness rejecting transfusion or a Christian Scientist rejecting surgery – the shift is to the *must not* category regardless of the canons of good science. In the more usual case, the categories into which a recommendation falls may shift several times in the course of the illness.

For one person, a lipoma, acne or sebaceous cyst is something to be ignored; for another, it is a horrid blemish, so emotionally disabling that it demands removal. For this person *may* becomes *must.* For an elderly man or woman chemotherapy of disseminated cancer may mean a few months more of life, less pleasantly lived. For this patient, a *should* or *may* becomes a *must not.* For another person, the few extra months to do some essential things may make the rigor of treatment worthwhile. For still another, mild depression, anxiety or headache is tolerable, and can be coped with without resort to daily medications; to another, as the twenty-four million Americans daily taking mood modifiers will attest, even slight anxiety must be treated (Chambers et al. 1975, 141).

In making the "right" decision for an individual patient then, personal, social, economic, and psychological characteristics of the patient must be factored in. They clearly may modify, or even nullify, the scientifically cogent or logically consistent answers to the questions of what can be wrong? And what can be done? Here, where we are closest to the end, the *telos*, of the whole process, scientific modes of reasoning and scientific reasons are least pertinent, and indeed must be submitted to drastic revision in consideration of the patient's value choices.

The reasoning at this stage is mainly dialectical, ethical, and rhetorical. Physician and patient together must clarify the relationship of one recommendation with its opposite and weigh the reasons for each action. The ethical nature of the discourse at this point is obvious. Conflicts in the obligation of patient and physician to each other must be resolved before a "right" action can be settled upon. Where these conflicts are fundamental, the medical relationship may even be severed by either party, to be resumed with another physician.

Once the ethical and logical possibility and "strength" of arguments for one action over another are assessed by dialectic, then the reasoning becomes "rhetorical" – in the more classical sense of artful persuasion, of relating a dialectically established decision to prudent action, generating belief of another kind from scientific or logical cogency, belief that this particular action should be taken in preference to all others (Tversky 1972, especially 27–28).

We enter here the delicate realms of how much persuasion is ethically defensible, how vigorously the physician should pursue his/her own priority system. Does he/she believe the scientifically recommended action must take priority? Is he/she a therapeutic enthusiast who prefers to "do something" rather than nothing? Does he/she think people should be "strong" and ignore minor infirmity?

Likewise, the patient can use artful persuasion to modify the physician's scientific or dialectically secured recommendation to gain an action more congenial to his/her view of what is good. The patient's vulnerability can easily tip the resolution of conflict in the physician's favor. But these are subtle influences, as well, which can significantly shape the physician's final judgment. The last question in the sequence then – what should be done? – the capstone question, as it were, which completes the whole structure, is the most prickly. Scientific and semi-scientific conclusions of varying degrees of certitude are examined under a light strongly tinged with moral hues. The accessibility of the questions to scientific modes of reasoning declines, as does the degree of certitude, as we move from determining what is wrong. To what *can* be done, to what *should* be done. The optimization of several kinds of uncertainty remains a central concern even when the conclusions are scientifically defensible.

The intermingling of several modes of reasoning – clinical scientific, probabilistic, dialectical, rhetorical and ethical – does not suggest immunity from explicit statement nor deprecation of attempts to secure truly scientific conclusions. But, it is warrant for setting limits on the utility of any of the current explanatory models – scientific, probabilistic, Bayesian, judicial simulation, decision analysis, inference, information or catastrophe theories. Perhaps the fullest explication will come from some combination of these new theories and more classical modes of reasoning.

11.4 Projection of the End of Right Action on the Process of Clinical Judgment

We have seen that clinical judgment requires confrontation with three generic questions which end in a particular decisive action for a particular patient. Several interdependent reasoning modes are requisite and suitable to each question, and no one question is entirely isolable from the others. We are ready now to turn briefly to a more specific delineation of how the end of right action projects itself upon the way the questions are answered. We might accordingly label this section "clinical prudence" – or, medicine viewed as a virtue.

Whenever possible, the clinician will try to achieve diagnostic closure, i.e., satisfy all the stringent criteria for certitude in locating his/her patient precisely in a classificatory schema. This is the admirable aim of scientific medicine; it is the ideal taught in academic settings; the more it is achieved, the better foundation there will be for the decision to act, at least some uncertainty will be eliminated.

Many clinical realities can upset the orderly processes of diagnostic reasoning: the urgency of the patient's condition, the absence of a diagnostic set or algorithm which fits the presenting signs and symptoms closely enough, lack of specific tests to discriminate among probable diagnoses, incomplete or inconclusive probability estimates, limitations on data selection related to cost or geographic locale, unreliability of the patient as historian, and the dilemma of weighting the probability of a serious vs. nonserious, and treatable vs. nontreatable disorder, when none of these possibilities is definitely excludable.

Experienced clinicians deal with these commonly occurring inevitabilities with interpretative schemata, which enable them to act prudently on inadequate information and incomplete evidence. These schemata can be loosely regarded as rules of clinical prudence, empirically derived but certainly not mysterious sources of inspiration. We can examine a few of these (Fig. 11.5).

SOME RULES FOR CLINICAL PRUDENCE

1. ACT TO OPTIMIZE AS MANY BENEFITS, MINIMIZE AS MANY RISKS AS POSSIBLE.

2. THE SERIOUS AND TREATABLE MUST NOT BE MISSED; THE NON-SERIOUS AND NON-TREATABLE MAY BE MISSED.

3. USE THE CLINICAL OCKHAM'S RAZOR: DON'T MULTIPLY CAUSES, DISEASES, TESTS OR TREATMENTS WITHOUT JUSTIFIABLE NECESSITY.

4. "REST" THE CASE FOR ANY DIAGNOSIS OR TREATMENT WITH RELUCTANCE.

5. CLINICAL SKEPTICISM IS THE ONLY GUARD AGAINST THE TYRANNY OF THE "ESTABLISHED" DIAGNOSIS, OR ANCILLARY DATA, AND THE FINDINGS OF COLLEAGUES (LAB, X-RAY, ETC.).

6. MAINTAIN A HIGH INDEX OF SUSPICION FOR UNCOMMON MANIFESTATIONS OF THE COMMON.

7. "HOOFBEATS DON'T MEAN ZEBRAS," UNLESS ZEBRAS ARE IN THE VICINITY.

8. WHEN THE DATA ARE "IN," CONTINUING DEBATE IS THE SAFEGUARD AGAINST ERROR.

9. RECOGNIZE YOUR OWN CLINICAL STYLE, PREJUDICES AND BELIEFS ABOUT WHAT IS "GOOD" FOR PATIENTS.

10. BE WARY OF HUNCHES, INTUITIONS, E.S.P.--GAMBLE WITH YOUR OWN FATE, NOT THE PATIENT'S.

Fig. 11.5 Some rules for clinical prudence

For one thing, the clinician thinks not so much of meeting the criteria for diagnostic closure, but how much evidence is "enough" to take an optimizing action. Diagnostic closure for example in streptococcal pharyngitis might demand sore throat, plus cervical adenopathy, tonsilar exudate, and positive culture for Beta hemolytic streptococcus. The physician is justified in giving specific treatment with penicillin on any combination of these signs and symptoms and positive culture. But he/she usually acts presumptively – taking a culture, treating, and awaiting the culture to determine whether to continue or discontinue penicillin. If the patient, however, lives in a family or school in which streptococcal illness is frequent or currently present, the most minimal clinical signs may justify treatment even without culture.

Acute abdominal pain is another example. It may result from a wide variety of conditions all of which can present similar signs and symptoms. Examples are: ruptured peptic ulcer, appendicitis, twisted ovarian cyst, strangulated internal hernia, mesenteric adenitis, pancreatitis, cholecystitis. Some of these conditions require immediate surgery, some delayed surgery, some none at all, and in some surgery is positively dangerous. The surgeon looks not for definitive diagnosis but for the least signs of acute abdomen – spasm and rebound – which justify laparotomy. Only in this way can he/she assure that the treatable lesion is not missed. Each surgeon is allowed a certain number of normal appendices or negative explorations, provided he/she has *no* cases in which lifesaving surgery is missed.

In every branch of medicine, there are disorders for which specific and dramatic treatment or genuine cures exist. They must not be missed. They shape the diagnostic process very often out of proportion to their probability in a given case or in the general population. Some are rare like pheochromocytoma; some relatively rare like parathyroid adenoma; some are rare only in a particular locale like malaria or actinomycosis or blastomycosis. Still others were once common, but now infrequent, though still important like syphilis, malaria or diphtheria.

The clinician's attention therefore may not be focused on getting all the information needed to fill out the most probable classificatory set in its entirety. Rather, more emphasis is placed on the information he needs to take decisive action, or to "rule out" the conditions which in the interest of the patient's safety must not be missed. The clinician must find justification for his/her actions, therefore, in terms of what is right and prudent for the patient. If a serious treatable disease cannot be adequately "ruled out," therapeutic trial may be used as a diagnostic maneuver, i.e., specific treatment is undertaken for the serious disorder, and diagnosis arrived at indirectly by observing the effect. Such a course of action may be taken justifiably even if the probability of a less serious, nontreatable disease is much higher.

A corollary principle, which to some extent balances the search for the treatable and serious, is the admonition "don't look for zebras when you hear hoofbeats." This is a precaution against accepting the rare and esoteric even if the symptom complex is suggestive. Obviously, one cannot justify missing the more common, or losing the more unusual manifestations of a common disorder in the search for the curable but esoteric. Of course, on the African plain, hoofbeats do mean zebras and not palomino ponies or quarterhorses.

Equally influential is the clinician's Ockham's razor – "plurality of causes and diseases is not to be assumed without necessity." Clinicians, particularly in the clinicopathological conference, are conditioned to seek unitary explanations of signs and symptoms. This is another of the organizing principles which become part of the projective schema used by clinicians to select, screen and weigh data and to justify their decision. The same advice is salutary in therapeutics – the rule of therapeutic parsimony states that treatments must not be multiplied without necessity.

Another rule of prudence is the cultivation of a "high index of suspicion" – another quasi-rational way to cope with uncertainties and avoid "missing" something. Clinicians who follow this rule are unusually sensitive to the most minimal criteria for a diagnosis. They use that sensitivity to open up previously unsuspected possibilities or challenge what appears to be a more firmly established diagnosis.

Indeed, the most dangerous ground for clinical judgment is often not in making a new diagnosis, but in maintaining an index of suspicion high enough to challenge what appears to be an established diagnosis. Physicians, like all humans, tend to rest their cases if no contrary position challenges it. They become locked into or even enamored of the patient's classification, which can render them unresponsive to the most obvious signals of a new disorder, or an original diagnostic mistake. The more prestigious the original diagnostician or institution and/or the more respect one has for the colleague who has made the diagnosis, the more seductive is this error.

Skepticism is, as Santayana so mordantly said, the "chastity of the intellect" – and an indispensable attribute of the prudent clinician is an untiring skepticism about every aspect of a diagnosis or treatment. Perhaps the greatest failing of the contemporary clinician is an overadulation for laboratory and x-ray data fed in by specialists, whose techniques grow more arcane and also more potent daily. Far too often, a right action is justified by the uncritical acceptance of a chemical determination, a biopsy or an x-ray examination.

I do not intend to provide here a complete primer of clinical prudence. These few principles derived from experience illustrate how the intensity of the clinician's concentration on the end – a good decision for his/her patient – provides a projective schema which shapes every step on his way (Abercrombie 1974).

Projective schemata are, of course, individualized and personalized. They summate what a particular physician holds to be "good" medicine. Which rules of thumb are selected, why, and how, are fascinating questions still very much open to logical and psychological examination. A whole series of attitudes of mind, logical and epistemological assumptions, are combined to make up a clinician's diagnostic and therapeutic "style," just as genuinely as the way word and phrase are used to make up a writer's style. The clinician's "style" is really a statement of the reasons he/she will accept as justification for a particular action, for setting aside certain probabilities, or for earnestly persuading a patient to take one course rather than another, equally earnestly propounded by his/her colleagues.

Are these not the elements of the "art" of medicine, and are they not closed to precise analysis, the way the style of Horace or Camus is closed? I think not. I agree with Claude Bernard's comment in warning against sole reliance on clinical instinct and clinical sense.

Everyone knows in fact that habit may give a kind of empirical knowledge of things sufficient to guide practitioners. Even though they may not always be able to account for it at first. But what I blame is willfully staying in this empirical state and not trying to get out of it. (Bernard 1927, 203).

Each clinician's rules of prudence need more precise statement. Many are held in common by all good clinicians. Their utility or fallacy can and must be better studied. Most theoreticians have concentrated on the *normative* aspects of clinical judgment. We need to know more about the descriptive nature of the process – who uses what justifications, and how do they benefit or imperil the outcome for the patient? How much difference in mortality, disability, side effects, costs is there between a good and a poor decision maker?

Some physicians are therapeutic enthusiasts. They treat more often than not; they require less justification for using a medication than parsimonious therapists, who insist on demonstrable evidence of effectiveness and frown on the use of placebos or chemical coping for minor disorders. How much of "style" is simply peer conformity, personal intolerance of ambiguity, an obsessive compulsion to "prove" the diagnosis, or satisfy some idealized notion of what constitutes clinical "science"? Much of the cost of medical care, and even its outcome and satisfaction for the patient can turn on how the clinician plays the "game" of clinical judgment.

The psychological components in different reasoning styles are coming under closer investigation (Sokal 1964; Elstein 1976). We also need more extensive empirical descriptions of the reasoning habits of "good" and "bad" clinicians. What is the effect on outcome of different habits of reasoning? Which ones are crucial, which incidental and which positively deleterious? In this era of concern for the quality of care, answers to these questions cannot be avoided for very long.

There remain, to be sure, certain features of clinical judgment which for the moment seem closed to explicit analysis. Clinicians have their undeniable moments of sudden insight and discovery. Some clinicians are more consistently accurate in their insights than others. What does happen at that precise moment when the clinician decides that there is "enough" information to "make" a diagnosis or "take" a decisive action? Or, when a set of signs and symptoms suddenly "assembles" itself into a new classificatory pattern? Or, when a patient's clinical features suddenly "fit" a previously described pattern; or, when the precise datum which will answer a puzzling question is suddenly identified?

There is no reason to suspect that clinical diagnosis is unique in this regard. The phenomena of "insight" and "discovery" are common to scientific and nonscientific endeavors. Polanyi and Lonergan have attempted to describe the deep epistemological structures and relationships which permit the leap from the obvious and the known to the previously unknown. Polanyi holds that scientific knowledge is never wholly explicit but resides in tacit understanding which provides the belief which makes thinking about a truth possible. Lonergan links belief to immanently generated knowledge. Polanyi's "discovery" and Lonergan's "insight" are likened by their authors to the "Eureka" of Archimedes (Kroger 1977).

To what extent these epistemological notions can account for the obscure features of clinical reasoning is problematic. What must be avoided is the easy appeal to some special illumination peculiar to clinicians. To resort to terms like "art" or intuition is to impede explication of a socially significant process. Whatever name we use to subsume the indefinable elements in the process, the effort to explicate them further is a moral as well as intellectual responsibility.

This warning against subjectivism is consistent with a major thesis of this essay – that the nature of the end projects itself on the steps leading up to it. Everything in medicine ultimately is judged by its end – the healing of a patient – even those steps we think most immune to pre-logical or subjective interpretation like pattern definition and recognition. In defining a disease pattern, for example, we must choose among an infinite set of properties – signs, symptoms, tests, etc. That resultant pattern is useful only if it includes a finite, and manageable number of characteristics. In making the finite selection we apply a test of utility, related to the purpose of the pattern definition. That purpose is making a "right" decision for a particular patient.

In pattern recognition, the selection is similarly shaped by the end. We seek sufficient congruence with the pattern characteristic of the more serious or the more treatable disorder. We select in favor of patterns which optimize the decision for the patient even though they may be less defensible by the rules of logic or probability.

Statisticians, logicians and engineers can help the clinician to apply criteria of validity to the characters he/she selects and to manipulate the sets once they are defined. But these aids are of limited use without definition of the purpose for which the classificatory set is to be used. Sokal, a pioneer in mathematical taxonomy, recognizes that in medicine we may limit ourselves to fewer characters than might be taxonomically desirable because we want those most pertinent to decisive action for a patient (Schwartz et al. 1973).

Projective schemata shaped to the practical end of decision making are to a significant degree subjective. But they do not provide warrant for a wholly subjectivist interpretation of clinical judgments. The schemata can themselves become objects of critical scrutiny. We can in fact often judge whether a clinical diagnosis, treatment or decision is the right one by the outcome for the patient. The test of reality is always there in medicine, and it sharpens and corrects the projective schema, and the values assigned in each of the more formal inferential steps. It is as Ernan McMullin said of the interpretive schemata of science which contemporary philosophers of science have adduced to counter the ultra-objectivism of logical positivism:

> But what must be emphasized is that the skills of interpretation that help bridge the gap between the formalism of inference and the subjectivism of sheer personal assertion are themselves continually responsive to the demands of the objective order (McMullin 1974).

In medicine we have more immediate and dramatic verificatory possibilities than in many other sciences (death, recovery, disability, complication, dissatisfaction). We can aim realistically therefore to reduce to a minimum the residuum of indefinable elements in each step of the process of arriving at clinical action. This applies even to the more subtle nuances in style which distinguish superior from merely average clinicians.

11.5 Some Theoretical and Practical Implications

Clinical judgment is what physicians do that most clearly distinguishes their enterprise from other human activities. If there is to be a theory of medicine therefore, an understanding of clinical judgment must be a central element – though certainly not the whole of such a theory.

This essay has argued two major theses which bear on a theory of medicine: that clinical judgment is justified and defined by its end – a decisive action for a human in distress and that different kinds of reasons, and reasonings, are appropriate to the formulation of a "right" end.

There are several important implications for a theory of medicine or at least its prolegomenon as well as medical education. Only two of these will be examined briefly: (1) Is medicine a science, art, or virtue or all three; (2) What information should a physician have?

(a) *Medicine – science, art or virtue?*

Sober has, in this conference, summarized the arguments on both sides of the art-science controversy and they need no repetition (Sober 1978). He firmly identifies clinical reasoning with scientific reasoning. On the view we have proposed there is no question that significant parts of the process do fit both the classical and modern descriptions of a science.

Deductive, inductive and retroductive inference are used to evaluate, interpart and explain clinical observations. Hypotheses are tested by further observation, experiment and measurement, and reliability, accuracy and standardization of data are sought, if not always achieved. These criteria of the scientific method are most clearly pursued in making the diagnosis and selecting and evaluating treatments. Medicine is even more convincingly a science when it seeks explanations of clinical phenomena, in theories and mechanisms of disease. Medicine then fits Einstein's definition of science as:

> … the century-old endeavour to bring together by means of systematic thought, the perceptible phenomena of this world into as thoroughgoing an association as possible. To put it boldly, it is the attempt at the posterior reconstruction of existence by the process of conceptualization. (Chambers et al. 1975, 24).

But the principal aim of medicine, its distinguishing feature, is not the explanation of clinical phenomena, useful as this may be in raising the clinician's enterprise above empiricism and technicism. Explanations in Einstein's sense are the proper business of the sciences basic to medicine, but they are not synonymous with medicine. Medicine exists as medicine only when it engages in the full range of activities which constitute clinical judgment and which lead to decisive action in the interest of a particular patient.

In its complete expression as medicine, the clinician's enterprise embraces non-scientific as well as scientific reasons and justifications. This essay alludes to the dialectical nature of differential diagnosis, the ethical construction in deciding what is "good" for this patient, and the rhetorical dimensions in the mutual persuasion essential to a decision taken jointly by patient and physician. These latter are skills traditionally imparted by the liberal arts and humanities. They may be exercised in medicine on data validated by scientific method. While dependent upon the reliability of these data, medicine is not identical with the means whereby they are validated.

Is medicine then in any sense an art? Not as the term is used in the current art-science controversy. We have argued that clinical judgments must not be assigned to realms of the intuitive and ineffable which find their source in a presumed special intellectual light possessed by clinicians. I would prefer to reserve the word art in medicine to the perfection of the things done by the physician – the craftsmanship without which the decisions taken would be improperly, unsafely or clumsily done. The art of medicine lies in the degree of perfection each clinician exhibits in history taking, physical examination, performance of manipulative techniques like surgery and various diagnostic maneuvers – the work done.

These must not be mindless activities. They are a tekné in the classical sense – knowing what to do, how to do it, and why one does it. Art and tekné were synonymous in Aristotle and both involve reasoning,"... art is identical with a state of capacity to make, involving a true course of reasoning" (Aristotle 1940, *Met.* VI, 4, 1140a, 10). Aquinas, extending the Aristotelian notion called art a recta ratio factibilium, thus distinguishing it from science, a recta ratio speculabilium and prudence, a recta ratio agibilium. The undeviating determination of the work to be done (art) is distinguished from the undeviating determination of what is to be known (science) and the undeviating determination of the act to be done (prudence) (Maritain 1949, 7, notes 4 and 5; Aquinas n.d.).

If we carry this distinction a trifle further medicine becomes not only science and art, but also the virtue of practical wisdom – "... a true and reasoned state of capacity to act with regard to the things that are good or bad for man" (Aristotle 1940, *Met* VI, 5, 1140b, 5–6). Aquinas expanded the Aristotelian concept somewhat. He argued that, while art gives the capacity to reproduce a good work it does not assure that the product will be used for a good end. That remains to the virtue of prudence – "Consequently, prudence which is right reason about things to be done, requires that a man be rightly disposed with regards to ends" (Aquinas n.d.).

In this sense then, medicine is both art and virtue. It is art since it is certainly concerned with the perfection of what it does – with the skills needed to make logically secure clinical decisions and to do the procedures decided upon. But it is also a virtue since it must make "right" choices about the ends and purposes for which the decisions and actions are produced. Medicine must not only perform well but act well, it must choose what should be done to heal a particular patient whose good is the true end of the whole activity.

Medicine is then all three – science, art and virtue synergistically and integrally united in the clinician's daily activities. To disarticulate one member of this triad from the others is to dismember medicine – the essential feature of which is the special relationship each holds to the other. When this happens one becomes a scientist, an artist or a practitioner, but not a physician. Clearly, any unitarian formalization of the clinician's activity is bound to be misleading, and to define a part of what constitutes medicine but not the whole of it.

(b) *What should a physician know?*

I have explored elsewhere the many meanings of the term medical humanism – which can so easily become a slogan for whatever version of intellectual or practical activities we wish to justify (Pellegrino 1974). Here it is only necessary to reiterate that medical humanism is both a cognitive and compassionate response to the person of the patient. It embraces humanism as a set of cognitive skills largely derived from the humanities and these are integral to the conception of medicine as science, art and virtue. Humane medicine – indeed moral medicine – requires that the physician understand the distinctions between these intellectual and practical activities, the kinds of reasons each may adduce, their limitations when applied to each other's realms, the different sources of their methodology and the different subject matter appropriate to each.

If there is any merit in these proposals, they should be reflected in what it is physicians are expected to know. If medicine is a science, and art, and a virtue (in the classical sense) – medical students will need a more explicit education in the non-scientific components of clinical judgment. The skills required for sound dialectical, ethical and rhetorical reasoning modes must be more explicitly incorporated into professional education – especially in the clinical contexts within which decisions for patients are being made. The liberal arts, and the humanities, even though they might have been presented in pre-medical studies, need vigorous refurbishment in medical education where it will become more obvious to the student that he *needs* the liberal attitudes of mind to function fully as a physician.

The liberal arts have a legitimate place in medicine, not as gentle accoutrements and genteel embellishments of the medical "art", or even to make the physician an educated man. Rather, they are as essential to fulfilling the clinician's responsibility for prudent and right decisions as the skills and knowledge of the sciences basic to medicine.

These are very good reasons for rein fusing the liberal arts into medical education in addition to, but not necessarily to replace, the liberal education in the universities. Premedical education is shallowly rooted for a variety of reasons: The pressure for admission to medical school converts non-scientific subjects into obstacles to be endured rather than essentials to an educated life. Similarly, the humanities may have become too specialized themselves to fulfill their functions as instruments of the liberal arts. Appreciation of the humanities may come more slowly than in the sciences – usually only after the young physician has had some experience of the moral nature of so many of his decisions. Then, the intellectual constraints of a life dedicated only to professional studies are only belatedly perceived. For all these reasons, the liberal arts and humanities are today being taught as part of a medical education in a significant number of schools (Pellegrino 1976b).

The full implications of the anatomy of clinical judgment for the philosophy of medicine cannot be examined further in this essay. Clearly a theory of medicine must account for this, the physician's most characteristic activity. Hippocrates was partially right to make medicine a natural science; Celsus to call it a conjectural art, and Osler, a science of uncertainty. Any theory of medicine must accommodate all these elements and in the special way demanded by the need to make particular decisions for particular patients. A theory of right thinking, right doing and right acting must then be related to each other. The theory of medicine must also be shaped by the end to which all medical activity points – a right healing action – for that is what defines medicine uniquely.

> It is a simple fact but almost universally ignored in modern thought that when one loses sight of the end of one's thought and action, the thought and action waver between fanaticism and futility. (Buchanan 1938, 174).

References

Abercrombie, M. L. J. 1974. *The Anatomy of Judgment*. London: Penguin Books.

Adler, M. J. 1927. *Dialectic*. New York: Harcourt, Brace & Co.

Aquinas, T. n.d. *Summa Theologiae* (Trans: W. P. Hughes), Leonine text, 1a 2ae, Question 57, art, 3–4.

Aristotle. 1940. *Metaphysics*. (Trans: W. D. Ross). Oxford: The Clarendon Press.

Bernard, C. 1927. *An Introduction to the Study of. Experimental Medicine*. New York: Macmillan.

Black, D. A. K. 1968. *The Logic of Medicine*. Edinburgh: Oliver & Boyd.

Buchanan, S. 1938. *The Doctrine of Signatures: A Defense of Theory in Medicine*. Paul, London: Keegan.

Cabot, R. 1916. *Differential Diagnosis*. Vol. 1, 19. Philadelphia: W. B. Saunders Co.

Chambers, E. E., J. A. Inciardi, and H. A. Siegal. 1975. *Chemical Coping: A Report on Legal Drug Use in the U.S.A.* New York: Spectrum Publ.

Einstein, A. 1974. *Out of My Later Years*. Secaucus, NJ: Citadel Press.

Elstein, A. S. 1976. Clinical Judgment: Psychological Research and Medical Practice. *Science* 194:696–700.

Feinstein, A. R. 1967. *Clinical Judgment*. Baltimore, MD: Williams Wilkins.

Feinstein, A. R. Forthcoming. The Haze of Bayes, the Aerial Palaces of Decision Analysis, and the Computerized Ouija Board. *Clinical Bio-Statistics* 39.

Feinstein, A. R., and C. K. Wells. Forthcoming. *Randomized Trials vs. Historical Controls: The Scientific Plagues of Both Houses*. Washington, DC: Association of American Physicians.

Jacquez, J. A., ed. 1964. *The Diagnostic Process*. Ann Arbor, MI: University of Michigan Press.

Jaeger, W. 1944. *Paideia: The Ideals of Greek Culture* (Trans: by G. Highet), Oxford, New York, III, 17–19.

Koran, L. J. 1975a. The Reliability of Clinical Methods, Data and Judgments, First of Two Parts. *New England Journal of Medicine* 293 (13): 642–646.

Koran, L. M. 1975b. The Reliability of Clinical Methods, Data and Judgments, Second of Two Parts. *New England Journal of Medicine* 293 (14): 695–701.

Kroger, J. 1977. Polanyi and Lonergan on Scientific Method. *Philosophy Today* Spring:2–20.

Ledley, R. S., and L. B. Lusted. 1959. Reasoning Foundation of Medical Diagnosis. *Science* 130:9–21.

MacIntyre, A. 1977. Patients as Agents. In *Philosophical Medical Ethics*, ed. Spicker and Engelhardt, 197–212. Dordrecht, Holland: Reidel.
Maritain, J. 1949. *Art and Scholasticism with Other Essays*. New York: Charles Scribner & Sons.
McMullin, E. 1974. Two Faces of Science. *Review of Metaphysics* 27 (4): 655–676.
McNeil, B. J., E. Keeler, and S. J. Adelstein. 1975. Primer on Certain Elements of Medical Decision–Making. *New England Journal of Medicine* 293 (5): 211–215.
Murphy, E. A. 1976. *The Logic of Medicine*. Baltimore, MD: Johns Hopkins Press.
Pellegrino, E. D. 1974. Educating the Humanist Physician: An Ancient Ideal Reconsidered. *Journal of the American Medical Association* 227 (11): 1288–1294.
Pellegrino, E. D. 1976a. Philosophy of Medicine: Problematic and Potential. *Journal of Medicine and Philosophy* **1** (1): 5–31.
Pellegrino, E. D. 1976b. Preface. In *Human Values Teaching Programs for Health Professionals*, ed. T. K. McElhinney, ix–x. Philadelphia: Society for Health and Human Values.
Pellegrino, E. D. 1977. Moral Agency and Professional Ethics: Some Notes on Transformation of the Physician–Patient Encounter. Commentary on Alasdair MacIntyre, "Patients as Agents". In *Philosophical Medical Ethics*, ed. S. Spieker and H. T. Engelhardt, 213–220. Dordrecht: D. Reidel.
Raiffa, H. 1968. *Decision Analysis: Introductory Lectures on Choices Under Uncertainty*. Reading: Addison-Wesley.
Schwartz, W. B., G. A. Gorry, J. P. Kassirer, and A. Essig. 1973. Decision Analysis and Clinical Judgment. *The American Journal of Medicine* 55:459–472.
Sober, E. 1978. *Learning Theory and Clinical Practice*. (in this volume), 29–44.
Sokal, R. R. 1964. Numerical Taxonomy and Disease Classification. In *The Diagnostic Process*, ed. J. A. Jacquez, 51–68. Ann Arbor: University of Michigan Press.
Tversky, A. 1972. Elimination by Aspects: A Theory of Choice. *Psychological Review* 79 (4): 281–299.
Weaver, R. 1968. *The Ethics of Rhetoric*. Chicago: Henry Regncry Co.
Wulff, H. R. 1976. *Rational Diagnosis and Treatment*. Oxford, England: Blackwell Scientific Publications.

Chapter 12
The Subjective in Clinical Judgment

Eric J. Cassell

12.1 Introduction

Someone telephones the doctor that he has had increasing dull pain in the right side of his abdomen and back for several hours. While not exactly nauseated, he is repelled by the thought of food. He thinks the pain is the same as that of his wife when she had her gallbladder attack. The patient's complaint is clearly subjective and of the type that most often initiates the medical act. Yet, in its subjectivity, the report lies in a domain of medical practice that is least understood, or more precisely that is least systematized. The deficiencies of medical practice in regard to the subjective are highlighted by the increasing use of the problem-oriented medical record as a tool of medical education. In *Medical Records, Medical Education, and Patient Care; The Problem-Oriented Record as a Basic Tool,* Lawrence Weed (1969) points out the equal importance of patients' subjective experience with objective, measurable facts of medicine. Further, Dr. Weed gives excellent examples of the kind of profiles of patients' personal and social lives that should be included in any complete medical record.

It has been my experience, however, that the problem-oriented medical record *as actually used* by the medical students and house officers at the New York Hospital (many of whom trained at other schools) is a sterile instrument that rarely meets the

This chapter originally appeared as Eric Cassell, "The Subjective in Clinical Judgment," in *Clinical Judgment: A Critical Appraisal*, ed. H.T. Engelhardt, Jr., et al. (D. Reidel Publishing, 199-215. Reprinted with permission from Springer.

Eric J. Cassell died before publication of this work was completed.

E. J. Cassell (✉)
New York, NY, USA

L. M. Rasmussen, S. Holm (eds.), *50 Years of Philosophy and Medicine*,
Philosophy and Medicine 150, https://doi.org/10.1007/978-3-031-95175-6_12

goals set for it precisely because it is deficient in its recording of the subjective. It has also been my experience that many younger (and too many older) physicians distrust the patient's report of his own symptoms and experience.

One more comment seems necessary to document the problem of the subjective in medical practice. The social medicine movement of earlier decades succeeded in establishing the importance of the patient's social and personal history as part of any complete medical record. And yet, a generation later that aspect of a patient's history is usually confined to personal habits (tobacco, alcohol, etc.), job history and some marital and family facts. The movement was successful in getting some aspects of the patient as subject into his own care but in a fashion often uselessly sparse because only the objective facts of the patient's existence are recorded.

12.2 The Subjective in Medicine[1]

I believe the subjective involves four aspects: the sociologic person, the unconscious, experiencer, and assigner of understandings. The sociologic person includes the patient's past and present cultural set, his roles (attorney, mechanic, father, son, etc.), the unfolding story of his life and his important others. The subjective also includes the unconscious self, generally considered to be conflicts, repressed materials, drives and motivations – matters not volitionally available to the conscious mind. Then there are the things experienced by the body or person of the patient. These may be objectively non-confirmable as in the instance of abdominal pain or objectively confirmable as in the instance of fever. In all instances, after the experience has passed it is non-confirmable, although subsequent objective evidence may allow it to be inferred. Lastly the subjective includes the meanings assigned by the patient to the experience and events he reports. This includes feelings evoked, beliefs about the nature of disease or illness as well as its causes, and extends to feelings, perceptions and beliefs about physicians and the world of medicine.

Obviously these four aspects of the subjective in medicine are not truly separate and cannot be made to remain separate except for purposes of explication, as I am doing here, and except for action as when the physician asks questions. Together they are the subject *in* medicine and the subject *of* medicine. They are, in other words, the patient.

Indeed it would be difficult, for example, to distinguish that part of the patient that assigns meanings from, say, the unconscious, or even from the perceiving experiencer. But I hope to show that these domains of the subjective can be kept apart, if only in action, well enough to serve the physician as he makes his diagnosis and treats his patient.

[1] This essay deals primarily with the subjective of the patient, not the physician. It is concerned with the subjective information that is obtained from patients, not with how that information is processed by the doctor.

12.3 The Sociologic Person

Two domains of the subjectivity of the patient have received the most attention in medicine: the sociologic person and the unconscious. There is ample evidence that the sociologic person is important in medicine. Diseases as disparate as tuberculosis and coronary heart disease are influenced in their occurrence by the life history of the person who has them. The malnourished black child from a large ghetto family has a much higher probability of acquiring tuberculosis than the white suburban child of a Bell Telephone supervisor, especially if there is an old person with tuberculosis in the crowded ghetto apartment. And the Bell Telephone supervisor has a greater probability of dying of a myocardial infarction than the unemployed father of the black child, especially if the supervisor smokes cigarettes, is sedentary and has a family history of coronary heart disease. Modern medicine has made much of the contribution of sociological variables to disease production (although even Virchow was politically radicalized by his awareness of the contribution of social factors to typhus prevalence in Silesia). But while probabilities may be crucial to directing the diagnostic thinking of a physician, probabilities are often not as necessary in making a diagnosis as what the sick person *says*. More important, however, is that probabilities are objective parameters of the sociologic person, not subjective. The probabilistic person is seen as propelled towards his expected pattern of disease by facts of his existence which he (usually) did not create and over which he (often) has no control. In other words it is not that the sociologic person cannot be construed as a part of the subjective domain of medicine – part of the domain of the consciousness of the patient, but rather that its current use by medicine is primarily in the objective domain: measurable or at least objectively confirmable personal facts linked to confirmable facts about the lungs or the coronary arteries. Even Weed's use of the subjective in the profiles of patient examples is aimed towards useful objective information. This kind of information might help in the interpretation of other diagnostic information (in the sense that "divorced women with young children are often…" and so on). But such data, while undoubtedly helpful and even often vital in clinical decision making, are part of the subjective of the physician more than of the patient. Sociologic parameters do not tell us about *this* divorced woman, but rather about the class of divorced women. In a sense the use of these facts to speak for the person so much occupies the physician's head (not to say his or her preconceptions) that they prevent the physician from hearing what *this* divorced woman has to say.

12.4 The Unconscious

The other aspect of the subjective that has received widespread attention in medical practice is the unconscious. It is fair to say that one of Freud's major contributions to medical practice was to put the person as subject back into medicine. It is not necessary to detail the evidence to support the belief that there are unconscious determinants of symptoms and disease. The widespread acceptance of psychosomatic medicine is an acceptance of the influence of the mind on the body. Oddly, it is conceived of as the influence of the *unconscious* mind on the body: a mind not available to the volition of the person and almost always conceived of as causing illness or symptoms. It is somewhat interesting, if only historically, that this view maintains the Cartesian duality but gives the (separate) mind some control over the body. This view of the duality is not nearly as meaningful or useful as the view of mind and body as a polar duality discussed by Guttentag (1969). Much as North and South cannot exist without each other and mutually influence each other, so also do mind and body. Of more immediate importance to our discussion is that the way the unconscious domain of the subjective is most often used in medical practice excludes the subject. That is to say, the patient is seen as not knowing what his unconscious contains or is doing. It is not under the patient's control and even the patient's words are an untrustworthy guide to its contents and its actions. We, the physicians, take it that we know better than the patient what are the unconscious determinants of his symptoms or his disease. While that may well be the case, it is an uncharitable view of the patient since that view bypasses the consciousness of the patient just as effectively as does the dominant view of the sociological person.

To view the unconscious as solely an inaccessible domain with only negative effects on the body is also, I believe, an uncharitable view of the unconscious. This is not the place (nor am I the person) to attempt a summary of the various views of unconscious process. Nonetheless, it seems important to point out that any such summary would have to include the understanding that the patient's unconscious is part of his subjective aspect that is able to communicate to another person. And, the unconscious and its communication are legitimate expressions of that person. Unconscious communications are not merely unsuspected leaks of inadequately repressed material but purposeful expressions. As the unconscious can speak, it can also be spoken to (Harley 1967). Finally, and of more direct importance to medicine, the unconscious appears able to communicate with the body. These phenomena which can be glimpsed in biofeedback techniques, hypnosis and certain yoga feats suggest a relationship of the subjective person to the body that is at present minimally understood.

Thus, just as the sociologic person is often used and viewed in medicine as an objective thing apart from the consciousness of the patients, so too is the unconscious used and viewed. For both sociologic person and unconscious, such understandings tend to diminish the potential importance to medicine of those aspects as factors of subjectivity.

12.5 Experiencer and Assigner of Understandings

I believe I am warranted, if only for methodological reasons, in making a distinction between the experiencer and the assigner of understandings within the subject. When the patient reported the dull pain in the right side of his abdomen and back, which he thought was similar to his wife's gallbladder attacks, he was actually reporting two distinctly different things: first, the *experience* of a body sensation; and, second, his *understandings* – the meaning attached to the body sensations. The assignment of understandings was on at least two levels; that the sensation was painful, and that it might be gallbladder disease. Considerable attention has been paid to the "subjectivity" of reports of pain, (for which, the way it is usually used, you may substitute the word "unreliability"). It has been shown that what patients say, or that their behavior in response to pain, is influenced by their ethnic group (Zborowski 1969). But that is merely another way of saying that the report of pain generally includes some kind of meaning to the patient. On the other hand, I do not know of studies which show that what some people call "pain," others label "itch" or "tickle." And that seems to be because what people call pain are sensations arising from a discrete group of nerve fibers called pain fibers. What is shown by differing reports of what is presumed to be the same kind of pain, is that valuation by the patient is part of the report. A seemingly different kind of the assignment of understanding is that which implies that the pain is from a gallbladder attack. Indeed, many patients when reporting their illnesses never tell of symptoms but simply use diagnostic terms. "First I got a cold and then it turned into bronchitis." Or, "last week I had a virus and then it started my colitis off."

The dominant voice of the patient with abdominal pain was the voice of the assigner of understandings (the pain is gallbladder disease) rather than the experiencer. And it is common to say that the patient's understanding might not be an accurate reflection of the meaning of his symptom. But meaning in whose terms? It must indeed be an accurate reflection of the meaning of the symptom to the patient (unless he is lying – the unusual case). Rather when we speak of the patient's understandings being inaccurate, we mean inaccurate by the doctor's standards. To dismiss the importance of the patient's understanding is to dismiss him as subject. After all, whatever the actual disease, its importance to the patient, even if it is fatal, will depend on how it meshes back into the subjective – the collectivity of his meanings. Thus, to deal adequately with the subject of the patient we must find within the patient's report of an experience two things: what is the matter in our terms, and who is the patient. Since the patient's report of an experience is so heavily influenced by his understandings, careful questioning about the report of the experience offers the opportunity of finding out about *both* the disease and the patient.

To understand the process of the assignment of understanding it may be useful to view it in the same manner that has been used to relate a speaker to what he says (Percy 1975). A speaker, in relating a sentence, is saying something about something; the speaker is thus the *coupler* between *what* he says, and what he says it *about*. Thus when the patient tells us about a symptom, he does the same thing. He is the *coupler* between the experience and his verbal report of the experience. As we have already seen, to assign language to the report is to assign meaning, and to give meaning is to give his understanding of the experience.

But it is obvious that the report of experience is not the experience itself and that the memories and sensations that constituted the original experience remain available for reinterpretation. This is not to deny that perception is to some degree guided by the assignment of meaning, and that what steps the patient takes to broaden his perception of an event – for example, taking his temperature, feeling his abdomen, trying to remember what was eaten and so forth – are also guided by the assignment of understanding. But, if the raw sense data of an experience remain available for re-interpretation, than a new coupler – the questioning doctor – can be introduced between what is *said* (the assignment of meaning), and what it is said *about* (the raw sense data of the experience). To put it another way, the doctor can insert himself between the patient as experiencer and the patient as assigner of understandings. This may seem a complicated way of saying that to obtain the story of an illness, the doctor asks the patient questions, but I think more is being said. Since by eliciting answers the physician is forced to continue to use the patient as coupler (someone saying something about something), how does he disengage the patient as assigner of understandings? The classic answer is that the physician offers (at least to himself) an alternative hypothesis. That is to say, if the doctor believes the man with abdominal pain does have gallbladder disease, he asks questions about the pain, its relationship to food, previous episodes, associated symptoms, and so forth, until he has enough evidence to support his tentative diagnosis. Or if such evidence is not forthcoming, he rejects that diagnosis, proposes (to himself) another diagnosis, and repeats the procedure. In doing this, he is using the same reasoning that will guide his physical diagnosis, choice of diagnostic tests or other diagnostic aids. If he is a good physician, he will use strict standards for hypothesis testing, and if he is a poor physician, he will use loose standards.

The classic picture I have just provided of the physician as *history taker* is inadequate for several reasons. First, the physician will only find what he already knows. Each case may flesh out his conception of the disease as the patient describes somewhat different expressions of symptoms, but he cannot find that for which he has no diagnosis. Second, he will miss in the patient's symptoms the unfolding process that the disease represents within the patient. Thus he will be held to basically static or structural views of disease rather than as a process occurring through time. After all, the patient, as the container of the memory of succeeding events influenced by the abnormality within him, is virtually the only source of information about such a process (reinforced by the physician's observation of the change in physical findings and laboratory tests over time). Third, in that classical method of questioning, the doctor will emerge knowing little about the person who has the disease, the subject of his work. The idiosyncratic differences presented by different patients are seen by some physicians as *obstructions* to the diagnostic process rather than as an inherent part of the diagnosis. Finally, the doctor will not learn how the person of the patient interacts with basic pathologic mechanisms to produce the illness that is *this* person with *this* disease.

I would like to expand somewhat on those four points in a somewhat different vein. The classic understanding of the physician taking a history from the patient by extracting those, admittedly subjective, facts of the illness in order to make a diagnosis of disease is deficient because it excludes the person from the diagnosis. It is by now cliche in medicine to speak of the importance of the "person of the patient" to diagnosis and treatment. We do not label as cliche the saying "a coin lesion of the lung is a carcinoma unless proven otherwise." Why is the former a cliche but the latter not? Because "treat the patient as a person" is more a wish than agreed upon necessity and does not rest on established facts and procedures which lead to a defined course of action. It is more an ethical imperative than a medical directive. I would like to point out, however, that the clinical expression of the primary diseases of our time, arteriosclerotic heart disease, hypertension, diabetes, degenerative joint disease, and perhaps the malignancies depend on the individuating characteristics of the patient. Further, in marked contradistinction to the infectious diseases or the surgical diseases, the patient is the primary agent of his own treatment. That is to say, the patient must change his life style or behavior and comply with often complicated treatment requirements. This was brought home to me the other day as I tried to discuss with a Chinese-speaking patient the use of insulin, diet, and exercise for the treatment of diabetes through an inadequate interpreter.

Contrary to directives based on analogy to the infectious diseases, what is needed are directives for obtaining information about the patient as person now necessary because of the change in the disease pattern and the preponderance of chronic disease. This involves some understanding, in methodological terms, of how understandings are assigned by the patient to the sense data of experience – the meaning of experience. An experience is given meaning along four planes, or conversely in reporting sense data, the patient modifies it to conform to his understanding along four planes. They are: (a) the space-time continuum – when and where things happened; (b) the assignment of value in relationship to other values of the self – the process of adjectivization; (c) the assignment of causality – where did the thing come from and what is it expected to do; and finally, (d) the relationship of the experience to previous experiences of the self or of significant others.

When patients feel pain, or experience fever, diarrhea and abdominal pain, they interpret it to themselves along those four planes. I believe that virtually no alien body sensation can go uninterpreted although the degree and complexity of the interpretation may vary widely – as in dismissing a twinge or conversely building a case for cancer on the twinge. What I am describing is a process in which the original body sensations can lead to interpretation which is followed by a search for other data in memory or at the moment that aids in, confirms or disconfirms the interpretation. In this process some sense information will be dismissed as irrelevant, and other sense data perhaps will be elevated in importance within the patient. The assigner of understanding (within the patient) takes a history from the experiencer (within the patient) in much the same manner that the physician questions the patient.

The importance of examining the various dimensions along which the experience is given meaning is not only that by so doing the physician will obtain a more accurate picture of the original experience, but also a more accurate understanding of the subjectivity of the patient.

12.6 The Space-Time Continuum

People seem to vary enormously in their ability to report details about the time and place (including place on the body) of experiences. In part, this appears to be idiosyncratic – some remembering in great detail events of the distant past and some assigning everything before yesterday to the hazy past. It is my impression that the future may be handled by different individuals in a manner similar to their handling of the past. Time and place are often related… "It must have been 1975 because that was the summer we were in New Hampshire." Time may be used as a mechanism of denial so that the events become difficult to recall because they cannot be located in time. In an opposite manner, "I remember it as though it were yesterday" becomes a means of maintaining the largeness of the event. Some handlings of time do not seem to be due to individual variation. Terribly threatening events that are remembered seem to remain, for most people, close in time – "that accident couldn't have been a year already." Similarly, a far future but bad prognosis is often handled as though the threat were immediate. In all of this time seems to be dealt with as though it were a spatial not a temporal dimension. The more important the event is considered the closer to the present self it is perceived. An understanding of this is important to the physician both in obtaining the history of an illness and in discussing prognosis, future therapies and so forth. A patient with a right-sided abdominal mass and fever was considered to have an ameboma because his symptoms started while on an Asian journey. In fact, however, the first episode of abdominal pain had started a month earlier in London but was attributed by the patient to carrying a heavy suitcase (to borrow from a later topic). Careful questioning that related times and places on the trip to body sensations produced the classic story of an appendiceal abscess. The original appendicitis, the relief of pain with its rupture, a few days of fever, then quiescence, followed by a return of fever, pain, and a perceived mass.

From what we know of the patient's subjective use of the time-space dimension in relating a story, we may be able to tailor our description of his future as we think it will happen. The basic point is that an objective outline of the future temporal relationships of a disease process will be necessarily reprocessed by the subjectivity of the patient in terms of his past use of that dimension. And that reprocessing influences the course of the patient's illness. For example, one patient with rheumatic heart disease, told that an operation will probably be required in two years, lives in constant and continuing dread of the surgery, behaving as though it is imminent. For another patient, saying that the medication he is taking now is to forestall an event that might occur many years in the future (as in the prevention of stroke or heart disease in hypertension) is the equivalent of removing any sense of the importance of the event and therefore of taking the medication. Thus, the objective time scale of a disease or a projected course of action provides *merely the language for time, only the patient's subjectivity can provide its meaning to the patient* and the meaning is what the patient will use to direct his actions and his fears. As with all the dimensions of the subjective, the person's subjective sense of time-space can change. Indeed, some changes in time sense from childhood to old age appear developmental but events in one's life also can produce change in an individual manner. "What my illness taught me is that I have to value each day."

12.7 The Assignment of Value

A second plane of subjectivity is the assignment of value to experience, or the process of adjectivization. Adjectives used by the inner assigner of understanding do not merely modify nouns such as for example pain, swelling, dizziness, or nausea, rather they give those experiences a value relative to other values of the self. A pain may be described as mild, or excruciating, uncomfortable or sore. One patient describes the pain as merely discomfort while for another patient the same kind of pain is unbearable. The assignment of value is both idiosyncratic and held in common. Certain kinds of pain, for example, pressure on a nerve root, will be described with the same kinds of adjectives by most people and this commonality allows adjectives to enter the diagnostic process much like an objective referent. On the other hand, the experience of the pain may be adjectivized differently. In this context, I can point out that physical behaviors such as writhing or grimacing, or conversely sitting stoically, add to the process of value assignment. For some people experiences are either black or white – things are terrible or simply fantastic. For others, things are more varied but the colors of their adjectives are always intense. Every experience, bad or good, is assigned a strong term. For others everything is subdued, nothing is fantastic, nothing is terrible. Pain may be awful but never terrible. Their weakened leg is not "useless" but "rather awkward." Their whole, near fatal illness was "a bore." The ethnic or cultural contribution to the assignment of value is well known.

The experiences of life enrich adjective use because these are values assigned relative to the other values of self. Since it is virtually impossible to speak without using adjectives, speakers quickly display their palette of value terms. On the other hand, many phrases or utterances do not include adjectives but their voice pitch, inflection and modulation emphasize or deemphasize the words, serving the same valuative function as the adjective in displaying the weight the speaker assigns to the words or thought. Consequently, as the physician obtains the story of an illness, he has available to him the scale of value assignment used by the patient. Consciously or not, those adjective usages and speech inflections (as well as clothes and body motion) allow him not only to understand the patient's value scale but also to revalue in his own terms the experience being reported. Similarly, since values are assigned relative to other values of the self, the physician has the opportunity to find out how important a symptom or possible consequence of an illness may be. Mild diminution in vision may be well tolerated by a patient who does not like to read but the same loss would be "intolerable" to an avid reader.

The pattern of valuings of a person is a basic constituent of that person. When the patient complains that something is "terrible" it is useless for the physician to say that it is not terrible. For the patient the thing is "terrible", "useless", "hopeless", "sad", "wonderful", "amusing", "interesting", "dirty", "smelly", etc. It is part of their understanding of the thing. And as it is part of their understanding of the thing, it is part of them as a person for we are constituted by our meanings and our meanings include the values we assign. For the physician to argue with his patient in order to change the valuing of something from "terrible", for example, to "mild" is not to change a word but the person himself. When two people look at a plate of six raw oysters one sees six oysters revolting and the other six oysters delicious. Induced to eat those oysters, a person may change his valuing of oysters from "revolting" to "delicious" because he has changed in regard to oysters. (The six remains a constant, however, and that is the infinite advantage of the number in the realm of value.) The patterning of value may change with experience and with that change comes a new understanding of experience and an alteration in the person himself.

This is an appropriate place to point out again that dividing the assignment of understandings into four planes and even separating these dimensions from the sociologic person or the unconscious is a useful procedural device for a physician but does not correspond to the person as he lives and thinks.

The person is a functional unity and these planes and dimensions interpenetrate. The assignment of value is heavily influenced by the sociologic person, by the cause of a symptom as perceived by the person (pain that is heart disease versus pain from a sore muscle), as well as by repressed unconscious material and even by the inner relationship of person and body. That these levels are a nexus rather than discrete does not detract, however, from finding out how a person assigns value. On the contrary, understanding how a patient assigns value is an important clue not only to the complete entity but to how the interpenetration occurs.

12.8 The Assignment of Cause

A third plane of subjectivity is the assignment of cause to the sense data of experience. No event can be experienced without a search for cause. I have called this the dimension of causality, rather than cause and effect, because as every event is understood in part by understanding its cause, it is also given meaning by a conception of what will follow from the event, in other words, what it will subsequently cause. As is the case with space-time and the patterning of value, understanding the cause of one individual event does not occur apart from the person's whole pattern of causal understandings. To believe that his pneumonia was caused by a bacterium or virus, the patient must conceive of micro-organisms as existing and as being part of the general class of causes. If that understanding exists, it may be applied by the patient to a whole range of phenomena experienced in his body. Thus, alien body sensations may be subsumed under their cause as in "I had a virus last week." The physician also has such a causal nexus but his understandings may be different. To him virus may mean for example coxsackie, varicella-zoster, or mumps virus in their most specific technical sense as well as a more general and vague sense he shares with the patient of viruses as a cause. This distinction should allow me to make clearer what I mean by cause as part of subjectivity. The mumps virus is in the physician's understandings, an objective technical thing having among other specific characteristics physical shape, and also a distribution among the population or in the tissues of the host. By that general class of cause called "a virus" no such specific virus is meant, although specific viruses remain the objective referent on which the subjective is based. Rather, the subjective allows experience to be classified and put at rest, so to speak. Causes within subjectivity such as "viruses" always have antecedent causes such as "I was run down", which may have its own antecedent such as "I was under a lot of strain" and so forth. Viruses, in subjectivity, are not considered serious and so they usually are not seen as causing other serious events. The important thing for this discussion is to realize that when the patient says "J had a virus last week", he is saying very little about the sense data of the experience but a great deal about his causal nexus. For the information to be meaningful in classic diagnostic terms, the doctor must inquire of the experiencer within the patient for the specific symptoms to which the understanding "virus" was applied. To accept that the word "virus" means to the patient what it means to the doctor may lead to serious diagnostic errors, as may acceptance of the patient's words "bronchitis", "sinusitis", "stomach upset", or what have you. (Those words contain not only cause but also value assignment and time-space information since they are often more specifically inclusive than "virus".) However, not to listen to those words and to hear only the specific sought after symptoms is also to miss valuable information about the person. The causal relationships tell not only how the patient views this illness, but how all illness may be perceived in terms of cause. The train of antecedents I suggested before may ultimately have led to some psychological conception of disease causality. In another person the ultimate nexus may be self-blame and sin. The first words of a patient of mine who was found to have a cancer of the breast were, "I knew it, I'm being punished." As it is useless to argue with people about their time-sense or valuations, it is equally useless to tell them that carcinoma of the breast is not punishment for illicit behavior. Rather, it is important to see the disease and its treatment within the causal network of the patient. And that network is revealed in the words of the patient when symptoms are related. The patient's conception of cause may have to be sought but to understand the subjectivity of the person (indeed the person himself) that search is as vital as the hunt for symptoms.

12.9 The Association of Experience

The fourth plane helpful in assessing the subjectivity of the patient is that in which an experience is given meaning by its association with the experiences of significant others. The patient has noted pain and stiffness in his fingers. The cause is not readily apparent – that is, he cannot remember doing something to the hand that might cause pain. His knowledge of the word includes the conception of arthritis, but, at age forty, he seems too young. His mother had arthritis, and remembering her, he concludes he also has arthritis. The experience of the mother appears to be dealt with as though it is part of his experience. Many other examples could be given to show the influence on the patient's assignment of understanding that is exerted by the experience of family. That a young woman with an elevated cholesterol interprets every pain in her chest as angina may seem reasonable to a physician since many of her relatives died at an early age of coronary heart disease. We find it reasonable because we know the relationship between familial hypercholesterolemia and premature coronary heart disease. While the patient may use those objective facts to support her fears, the fear is part of her subjective experience of her parents. For example, another person with normal blood pressure and headache worries always about stroke and we are not surprised to find that a parent died of a stroke. The fear of the patient that he has the disease of the parent is believed by many to arise from unconscious deter· minants such as unresolved oedipal conflict, or unresolved guilt. Such interpretations may be correct, but whatever the reason, patients behave in a manner suggesting that the experience of significant others is part of their own experience when they assign understanding to their own experience. Further, I am frequently surprised at how difficult it is to dislodge the patient's belief that he has the same problem as the parent even in the face of considerable counter-evidence. As the physical therapist was working successfully on her previously painful knees, the patient was sure the therapy would be useless because her mother had been crippled by arthritis. Two different lines of thought are suggested by these observations. The first is that subjectivity, the collectivity of meanings, extends beyond the physical confines of the person. Such a conclusion, which is neither new nor world shaking, achieves its importance in this context because when the doctor talks to the patient he generally acts as though he is facing a unique free standing individual. The physician does not see the continuity of the patient with the parents or siblings and neither may the patient. The continuity might not even be important if it did not so color the assignment of meaning to experience. But more striking, *that continuity tends to determine the experience.* It is in this area that the relationship of the unconscious domain of subjectivity to the assignment of understanding seems most obvious. The relationship to parents and other important people does tend to occupy the content of repressed or conflictual material making much of that content unavailable (except by inference), to even the most skilled questioner in the limited time available to the physician taking a history.

On the other hand much of the continuity of experience is available to the patient on reflection and so also is the patient's belief that the experience of significant others may determine his own experience even if he does not consciously know why that should be the case.

Where the physician obtains a family history he generally obtains facts of family disease, such as diabetes, as well as who is alive or dead and their ages and so forth. That the mother may have had diabetes influences the probability that the patient has diabetes but does not help in the diagnosis. On the other hand the fact that the mother had diabetes may have a great influence on how the patient interprets and reports increased urination or other symptoms of diabetes. It may have even more influence on how the patient behaves after he is told of his own diabetes. I should like to stress that this frequent clinical observation should not be confused with interpretations as to its psychological cause. The subjectivity of the patient influences not only the assignment and report of the meanings of an experience but the patient's interpretation of subsequent events in the illness. It cannot be overstated that the interpretations of the patient help determine the way the disease will be expressed in the patient and the patient's behavior towards the disease. Not only the symptoms but also the totality of meanings, and actions that follow these meanings, are the illness.

Another line of thought follows from these observations. Patients do not only borrow from the experience of family but also from that of friends and associates as they give understanding to their own experience. Physicians are sometimes frustrated to discover that the misinformation of friends or even casual acquaintances is given more weight by the patient than the doctor's knowledge. Why should this be? It seems to me that uncertainty is the primary impetus for the assigner of understandings. Uncertainty is intolerable. Where the previous experience or knowledge of the person is inadequate to give meaning to the events, others must be consulted. The fact that opinion from the unknowledgeable is influential cannot be because they lack knowledge, but rather because they have knowledge. But what knowledge can that be? I suspect that the associates have two advantages over the physician in the service of certainty. First, they *know cause* in the same terms as the patient, and second, the patient thinks they *know him* because they are like him. That is to say that the experience of the associates is useful in giving meaning to the patient's experience because the associates and the patient are similar. As one's subjectivity includes parents and siblings, it also includes the surrounding group. In providing their experience or knowledge the members of the group do two things: they give understanding to the events of the patient and they assure that what is happening to the patient does not exclude him from the group. The myths of the group are part of the subjectivity of the patient. It is often the case that the physician is not part of the group and further that his knowledge is seen as threatening whereas the knowledge of the group offers security.

12.10 Conclusion

For the purpose of understanding I have divided the subjective of the patient into (1) the sociologic person, (2) the unconscious, and (3 and 4) the experiencer and the assigner of understandings. Further, I suggested that understanding is assigned along four planes – (a) timespace, (b) value, (c) causality and (d) association. I think that the physician who is trained to hear in those dimensions will learn how the patient represents his symptoms to himself and assigns them meaning. But further the physician will also learn how the patient will understand future events including what the doctor will tell him of his illness. The patient does not have the option nor an *interest* in seeing things objectively, at least as far as his illness is concerned, because processing the sense data of experience *requires* the subjectivity of consciousness. Details of timing and causality and the adjectives that describe and modify the description of things to come only have meaning to the patient in his own spatiotemporal, causal and value terms. A month may have thirty days, but which is longer, thirty days of health or thirty days of pain caused by my own carelessness?

Two important things remain. First, my division of subjectivity is entirely artificial. Even for the purposes of understanding, these realms and planes should not be seen as parts of a whole. They are not like the muscles, nerves, blood vessels or bones of a limb–things in themselves. Perhaps at their most discrete they are reflecting facets of the whole, a way of beginning to know and appreciate the whole. To see them separately, to listen for them as the patient tells the story of his illness has methodological advantages since the person as subject is so hard to grasp as a whole. The pianist practices the concerto by working out parts of it until those segments are part of him sufficiently so that he can present the whole concerto to himself and then to others. I stress this because two previous attempts to get the subject into medicine represented by the unconscious and the sociologic person foundered because those aspects of person entered medicine as separate and unique entities. Nor have I said what in the person is the assigner of understandings. I do not know and I do not think it is necessary to know. It has been said that a spoken utterance is unique because it can mean literally anything. It achieves its meaning in the moment, the context of other utterances, situation and place and by who says it and who listens. Here also the meaning of events is relative. My divisions and planes of the subjective, as my colleague Dr. Skopek has pointed out, are merely schemes of relationships and in those terms are not totally artificial. But what in the person untangles the relationships is irrelevant.

Finally in this discussion, the interpreter of particulars of the subjective is the physician. Earlier I suggested the image of the physician interposing himself between the experiencer and the assigner of understandings. If he listens only to the sense data of the experiencer he will hear only about disease and will miss the person. If he hears only the subjectivity he will miss the disease. To listen to both without knowledge of disease and knowledge of persons is to miss everything. Have I assigned a role to the physician that I deny to the patient–the ability to keep separate his observation of what the patient says (including how he says it) from his own assignment of understanding or interpretation? Yes, I have done that because I believe that to make *use* of the subjective (rather than just to live it in the everyday) the physician must learn to separate his observation from his interpretation. A difficult task but one that can be taught and learned. We teach the same art in physical diagnosis because we know what we want the student to see and provide a schema with which to evaluate it. Then we hope he will go on to see not only what he has been taught but also, for example, how the skin looks and feels; how the patient walks and how he moves – the endless details of the visible body. The analogy to physical diagnosis is important because there, as in the subjective, we do not expect very much in the beginning. It is our hope, as teachers, that having provided the reason and the tools to see the body, time and the student's ability will enlarge both his knowledge and his views. With the subjective we can only do the same. Provide the reason and the tools to listen and then hope that the physician will hear the person much as the pianist first reads the music and practices individual parts of the concerto. The art of physical diagnosis, then laboratory diagnosis and even clinical thought itself has evolved over the years in a reciprocating relationship to knowledge of disease. The place of the subjective in clinical judgment has rested on intuition for too many centuries. But now it is emerging in response to the demand for a medicine of persons rather than a medicine of disease – a whole medicine, not merely a medicine of the body.

Acknowledgment This work was supported in part by a grant from the Henry L. Blum Research Fund and the Robert Wood Johnson Foundation. With the assistance of Nancy McKenzie.

References

Guttentag, O. E. 1969. Medical Humanism: A Redundant Phrase. *The Pharos,* January, 12–15.

Harley, J., ed. 1967. *Advance Techniques of Hypnosis and Therapy: Selected Papers of M H. Erickson*. New York: Grune & Stratton.

Percy, W. 1975. *The Message in the Bottle*. New York: Farrar, Straus and Giroux.

Weed, L. 1969. *Medical Records, Medical Education, and Patient Care; The Problem-Oriented Record as a Basic Tool*. Cleveland: Press of Case Western Reserve University.

Zborowski, M. 1969. *People in Pain*. San Francisco: Jossey-Bass Inc.

Chapter 13
What Is the True Death of a Human Being?

Jason T. Eberl

13.1 Introduction

There are several notable historical contributors to the "birth of bioethics," one of which is the report of an *ad hoc* committee of the Harvard Medical School (1968) that offered a re-examination of the definition of death, leading to the US President's Commission for the Study of Ethical Problems in Medicine and Biomedical and Behavioral Research (1981) to develop model legislation known as the Uniform Determination of Death Act [UDDA] (Jonsen 1998, pp. 238–244). The UDDA – subsequently adopted either verbatim or with limited modifications by every US state, district, and territory, and influencing additional legislation around the world – states that a human being's death may be legally declared utilizing either of the following criteria: "(1) irreversible cessation of circulatory and respiratory functions, or (2) irreversible cessation of all functions of the entire brain, including the brain stem."

Almost immediately following the publication of the Harvard committee report, debate ensued among medical practitioners and scholars within the nascent field of bioethics regarding the validity of the use of neurological criteria – typically referenced as "whole-brain death"[1] – to determine that a human being has died. Critics have generally gone in one of two directions: either calling for (a) adherence to the traditional circulatory/respiratory criterion alone – (1) in the UDDA – or (b) recognition that the death of a human being *qua* "person" occurs with the irreversible

[1] Though, for reasons specified below, a perhaps more accurate label would be "death of the brain as a whole" (Bernat 2019).

J. T. Eberl (✉)
Albert Gnaegi Center for Health Care Ethics, Saint Louis University, Saint Louis, MO, USA
e-mail: jason.eberl@slu.edu

L. M. Rasmussen, S. Holm (eds.), *50 Years of Philosophy and Medicine*,
Philosophy and Medicine 150, https://doi.org/10.1007/978-3-031-95175-6_13

cessation of neocortical functions alone – so-called "higher-brain death."[2] Defenders of whole-brain death have developed various *biophilosophical* rationales to justify its continued clinical use alongside the circulatory/respiratory criterion as stipulated by the UDDA.[3]

The debate concerning how to conceptually define and clinically determine a human being's death has thus been a central concern for the entire lifetime of the field of bioethics. At the root of this debate are several philosophical claims regarding, for example, the definition of human personhood and criterion of personal identity, operative concepts such as "organism as a whole" and "irreversibility," and the question of whether death should be understood as a strictly biological or a partially socially constructed fact. It was thus most appropriate for Springer's "Philosophy and Medicine" series to have taken up this topic with two volumes specifically devoted to it. The first volume, edited by Zaner (1988), responded directly to the President's Commission report and its formulation of the UDDA. It comprised essays that examined the questions at hand from historical, conceptual, legal, and cultural vantage points, including essays that not only critiqued the whole-brain criterion but also argued in favor of the neocortical criterion. The second volume, edited by Potts et al. (2000), followed the publication of a series of landmark articles by pediatric neurologist and brain death critic D. Alan Shewmon. The essays composing this volume are authored by physicians, philosophers, and theologians representing international perspectives from the U.S., U.K., Europe, and Japan.

A quarter-century later, the brain death debate has not waned and in fact has been re-energized by recent cases involving apparent post-brain death survival such as that of Jahi McMath (Aviv 2018), an attempt to revise the UDDA through the US Uniform Law Commission (Lewis et al. 2019, 2020), and the development of a novel means of organ procurement known as normothermic regional perfusion following determination of death by the circulatory/respiratory criterion (Bernat 2024; Busch 2024). It is thus time to revisit the arguments for and against brain death,[4] as well as arguments favoring the circulatory/respiratory criterion. In this essay, I will not only defend the conceptual validity of brain death, but also argue that brain death indicates the *true* death of a human being and that the circulatory/respiratory criterion is valid only insofar as it may also serve as a clinical indicator that brain death has occurred.

---

[2] For an example of the latter position, see Veatch and Ross (2016, Ch. 5). References to advocates of the former position will be provided below.

[3] I will discuss two representative biophilosophical rationales below.

[4] From here on, unless otherwise specified, any use of the term 'brain death' will refer to the *whole*-brain criterion. There is an unfortunate conflation of the term 'brain death' with both whole-brain and higher-brain criteria, as evidenced during discussions of the case of Terri Schiavo, who was in a persistent vegetative state for fifteen years but was not whole-brain dead (Bernat 2008a).

13.2 Biophilosophical Arguments for and Critiques of Brain Death

13.2.1 Bernat

James Bernat has offered the most thoroughly developed biophilosophical defense of brain death. He roots his justification of the brain death criterion in an understanding of death being related to an organism "as a whole," which refers to "that set of vital functions of integration, control, and behavior that are greater than the sum of the parts of the organism, and that operate in response to demands from the organism's internal and external milieu to supports its life and to maintain its health" (Bernat 1998, p. 17; cf. Bernat 2008b, Chap. 11, Bernat et al. 1981).[5] Nearly all parties to this debate accept some version of this concept; otherwise, if we stipulate that every last neuron in the brain must cease firing before we declare someone dead, we would have to abandon even traditional cardiopulmonary means of determining death and await the onset of putrefaction before declaring a human being to have died (Oderberg 2019).

Bernat (1998, p. 17, 1999) further defines the "critical functions" of an organism as a whole, the cessation of all of which is necessary and sufficient to constitute the loss of an organism's functional unity: "(1) vital functions of spontaneous breathing and autonomic control of circulation; (2) integrating functions that assure homeostasis of the organism … and (3) consciousness." Bernat (2001, p. 176) then shows how these critical functions are dependent upon the brain:

> A review of the critical functions of the organism as a whole reveals that they are subserved within the brainstem, hypothalamus, thalamus, and cerebral hemispheres. Respiration and blood pressure control are generated in the brainstem. The complex array of regulatory, feedback, and homeostatic mechanisms are integrated in the brainstem and hypothalamus. Consciousness requires the ascending reticular activating system of the brainstem, thalamus, and cerebral hemispheres. Therefore, the clinical functions of each major part of the brain must be absent for the cessation of the critical functions of the organism as a whole.

Bernat contends that the absence of these neural functions is not only *necessary* for a human organism's death, but also altogether *sufficient*. His three categories of critical functions that define the existence of an organism as a whole can be collectively termed the organism's "integrative unity." Bernat (2002, p. 334) concludes that the brain, as a whole, is an "irreplaceable, indispensable, complex, structural-functional control system that maintains the health and life of the organism, without which the organism no longer can function as a whole."

[5] For further articulation and defense of the concept of an "organism as a whole," see Bonelli et al. (1999).

13.2.2 Shewmon

As noted above, one of the most vocal and oft-cited critics of the any neurological criterion for determining human death is D. Alan Shewmon. A previous defender of both higher- and whole-brain death (Shewmon 1985, 1992), Shewmon planted his stake firmly in the anti-brain death ground with a quartet of seminal articles published in legal, medical, philosophical, and theological journals (Shewmon 1997, 1998a, b, 2001). Shewmon rejects the brain death criterion after examining cases in which a human body appears to maintain its integrative unity after whole-brain function has irreversibly ceased. Such cases lead Shewmon (2004, p. 38) to conclude that the brain does not function as the body's central organizer, but rather "fine-tunes" the vital functions that the body itself exercises as an integrated whole:

> The brain cannot be construed with physiological rigor as the body's "central integrator," in the sense of *conferring* unity top-down on what would otherwise be a mere collectivity of organs ... A living body possesses not an integra*tor* but integra*tion*, a holistic property deriving from the mutual interaction among all the parts.

If, as Shewmon argues, a body can maintain its integrative unity without any brain function, then brain death cannot be equated with a human organism's death. Shewmon (2007) thus favors the circulatory/respiratory criterion alone for determining when death occurs.

Shewmon (2001, p. 460) purports that a human organism, without a functioning brain, can have "at least one emergent, holistic-level property" and that the existence of any such property is sufficient for an organism to have integrative unity. Nicanor Austriaco (2003, p. 292) elaborates: "A property of a composite is defined as 'emergent' if it derives from the mutual interaction of the parts, and 'holistic' if it is not predicable of any part or subset of parts but only of the entire composite." To demonstrate that the requisite holistic-level property exists, Shewmon (2001, pp. 467–468) provides what he terms a "litany of non-brain-mediated somatically integrative functions" that have been observed to persist in the body of a brain dead individual. Such functions include homeostasis of various mutually interacting chemicals, cellular waste handling, energy balance, maintenance of body temperature, wound healing, infection fighting, stress responses, proportional growth, and even sexual maturation.[6]

Shewmon appeals to a number of cases in which a brain dead individual appears to exhibit integrative somatic functioning.[7] The most provocative cases involve patients who are properly diagnosed as brain dead and yet survive for extended

---

[6] Shewmon (1998b) offers a detailed analysis of 56 cases of whole-brain dead individuals with prolonged survival and persistence of these apparently somatically integrative functions; although he actually collected 175 cases in which whole-brain dead individuals survived at least 1 week (Shewmon 2007, p. 307). For an additional list of vegetative functions which may persist after whole-brain death, see Karakatsanis and Tsanakas (2002, pp. 129–133).

[7] The longest recorded case of somatic survival – 24 years – following brain death is known in the literature as 'T.K.' (Repertinger et al. 2006).

periods of time with technological and pharmacological support. Despite the requirement of mechanical ventilation for respiration and circulation of oxygenated blood to occur, Shewmon contends that these patients exhibit integrative unity by virtue of exercising the somatic functions listed above. He thus concludes that these patients cannot be considered dead, even though they lack brain function.

13.2.3 President's Council on Bioethics

In 2008, the US President's Council on Bioethics [PCB] published a white paper that provided, in light of Shewmon's challenges, an alternative biophilosophical foundation for brain death to the integrative unity rationale:

> Determining whether an organism remains a *whole* depends on recognizing the persistence or cessation of the fundamental vital *work* of a living organism – the work of self-preservation, achieved through the organism's need-driven commerce with the surrounding world. When there is good reason to believe that an injury has irreversibly destroyed an organism's ability to performs its fundamental vital work, then the conclusion that the organism as a whole has died is warranted (PCB 2008, p. 60).

This "vital work" rationale has been roundly criticized for, among other issues, implying that individuals who have experienced not only *whole*-brain death, but also *higher*-brain death, are no longer engaged in "need-driven commerce with the surrounding world" – despite the PCB explicitly rejecting higher-brain death – as well as insufficiently justifying spontaneous respiration as the *sine qua non* for an organism to be engaged in such commerce, eschewing all the other holistic-level activities Shewmon and others have previously identified as persistent in the bodies of whole-brain dead individuals (Shewmon 2009; Johnson 2016; Nair-Collins and Miller 2017). The PCB's "vital work" rationale, however, has been defended recently by Adam Omelianchuk (2021),[8] who calls attention to the need to consider the role neuroendocrine function plays in subserving an organism's "vital work" and the need to continually revisit the clinical diagnostic tests for brain death in light of cases such as that of Jahi McMath, to which we will now turn.

---

[8] For another defense of the "vital work" rationale as fitting with a phenomenological, as opposed to a cybernetic, understanding of organismic life, see Scherz (2022).

13.3 Recent Controversies

13.3.1 Jahi McMath

As discussed above, critics of the continued use of neurological criteria to determine death argue that moral certitude is lacking in light of purported evidence of persistent integrative unity of patients who have been declared brain dead and have yet vegetatively persisted for weeks, months, or even years. A recent case that sparked national controversy was that of a 13 year-old patient named Jahi McMath, who was declared brain dead following complications from oral surgery in Oakland, California. Her family did not accept that she was dead, however, and arranged to have her transferred to a long-term care facility in New Jersey, which allows for patients or families to conscientiously refuse brain death determination (Olick 1991). While some commentators warned against giving the family "false hope" (Caplan 2014), and it is the case that Jahi never recovered consciousness and her body ultimately succumbed to liver failure in 2018, others have questioned the accuracy of the initial brain death determination or have utilized her five-year somatic survival to challenge the validity of brain death altogether (Shewmon 2018; Shewmon and Salamon 2021).[9]

A significant issue highlighted by the McMath case, but well known for decades prior, is the "legal clinical mismatch" between what the UDDA requires for brain death to be declared and what is done in clinical practice, where testing for neuroendocrine function has never been required for determination of death (Robbins and Bernat 2020). A recent review showed a significant number of patients who met the criteria for brain death nevertheless had persistent hypothalamic and pituitary function and thereby did not meet the UDDA's requirement of "irreversible loss of *all* functions of the *entire* brain" (Nair-Collins et al. 2016; Nair-Collins and Joffe 2023). This issue has sparked disagreement among brain death proponents concerning whether testing for neuroendocrine functions, specifically those associated with the hypothalamus, should be added to the authoritative brain death assessment guidelines published by the American Academy of Neurology [AAN] (Greer et al. 2023).

Recognition of this discrepancy between the UDDA and actual clinical practice has led to diverse calls for revising the UDDA to bring the law and practice into alignment. In one direction are those who contend that testing for neuroendocrine function should be added to the AAN guidelines (Nair-Collins 2023; Sulmasy 2019; Sulmasy and DeCock 2023; Sulmasy et al. 2024). In the other direction are those who argue that the language in the UDDA referencing "*all* functions of the *entire*

[9] Another well-publicized case is that of Marlise Muñoz, who became brain dead while 14-weeks pregnant (Stevens 2014). Although Muñoz was eventually taken off of the ventilator prior to her fetus attaining viability, there have been several cases of brain-dead pregnant patients being ventilated until their bodies are able to birth a viable fetus (Bernstein et al. 1989; Field et al. 1988; Dillon et al. 1982).

brain" should be changed such that persistent neuroendocrine function is not a defeater for brain death determination (Lewis et al. 2019, 2020).

13.3.2 NRP-cDCD

Another change being sought by some proponents of revising the UDDA is to change the 'irreversible' requirement to 'permanent.' The rationale is another misalignment between what the UDDA legally requires for death to be declared and what occurs in practice – specifically, the process of organ procurement following circulatory determination of death. The current practice of controlled donation after circulatory death [cDCD] begins with a patient who is not brain dead but is being maintained by life-sustaining treatment such as mechanical ventilation.[10] A decision is made, either in accord with the patient's advance directive or by an appropriate surrogate decision-maker, to discontinue life-sustaining interventions and to donate the patient's organs. In standard cDCD, once life-sustaining interventions are discontinued, the transplant team waits for the patient's heart to stop beating (asystole), followed by a "hands-off" waiting period of usually 2–5 minutes to ensure that spontaneous heartbeat will not resume. At the end of this waiting period, the patient is declared dead and organ procurement begins. This practice purportedly accords with the "dead donor rule" [DDR], which states that organ procurement should never kill a patient and may begin only after the donor has been declared dead (Robertson 2000).[11]

A novel form of this practice involves maintaining the circulation of oxygenated blood using extracorporeal membrane oxygenation [ECMO] or cardiopulmonary bypass, known as normothermic regional perfusion with controlled donation after circulatory death [NRP-cDCD]. This process begins the same way as other cDCD procedures; however, following the declaration of the donor's death, the arteries that provide blood to the donor's brain are ligated in order to occlude cerebral circulation and, as the American College of Physicians [ACP] (2021) describes it, "to bring on brain death."[12] The donor is then connected to ECMO or a bypass circuit that

---

[10] *Uncontrolled* DCD [uDCD] occurs when a patient suffers spontaneous cardiac arrest and death is declared after the decision has been made to cease or not employ resuscitative efforts; uDCD is less practically feasible than cDCD for obtaining viable organs for transplant. For further details on DCD – formerly known as "non-heart-beating donation" – see the two reports from the Institute of Medicine (1997, 2000).

[11] For ethical analyses of the validity of DCD with respect to the DDR, see DuBois (1999, 2002) and Menikoff (2002).

[12] For a response to this ACP's statement, see Parent et al. (2022), which describes the intentionality behind the occlusion of cerebral blood flow as removing "doubt regarding any degree of coordinated neuronal activity" (p. 1308).

restores circulation and enables regional perfusion of the thoracic and abdominal organs.[13]

NRP-cDCD has illuminated what was already a "legal clinical mismatch" between what the UDDA requires and what is done in practice with respect to cDCD. Critics of such organ retrieval protocols contend that 2 minutes – or 5 or 8 minutes in more conservative protocols – is insufficient to ensure that spontaneous circulation cannot resume, and thus the *irreversibility* requirement has not been met:

> It is not clear that patients are dead within the first few minutes of apnea and asystole. It takes considerably longer than a few minutes for the brain and other organs to be destroyed from cessation of circulation and lack of oxygen. Moreover, it takes longer than this time for the cessation of heartbeat and breathing to be unequivocally irreversible, a prerequisite for death. As proof of this assertion, if cardiopulmonary resuscitation were performed within the first few minutes of cardiorespiratory arrest, it is likely that some of the purportedly "dead" patients could be successfully resuscitated to spontaneous heartbeat and some intact brain function (Bernat 1998, p. 20).

Although it would be quite rare for spontaneous circulation to resume without any resuscitative efforts, for many patients, if resuscitative measures were employed during the waiting period, spontaneous circulation could potentially resume. This potentiality evinces that the cessation of the patient's circulatory function is not, in fact, irreversible; rather, the resumption of circulatory function is prevented by the physician's decision – even if based on sound ethical reasons – not to employ resuscitative measures.

The practice of cDCD has led to calls to revise the UDDA to stipulate a requirement of *permanent* cessation of circulation following a decision to cease life-sustaining interventions and not to employ resuscitative measures once the patient's circulatory function ceases. Although the US Uniform Law Commission has to-date elected not to revise the UDDA in this way,[14] it is nevertheless a widespread practice to treat the permanent (by *fiat*) cessation of circulatory function as equivalent to such function being irreversible. Some philosophers have thus argued that we should reconstrue death not as a biological event determinable as an objective *fact* but rather as a complex constructed concept that involves not only biological realities but also social conventions regarding when it is appropriate to treat someone as dead (e.g., Lizza 2006).

Additionally, what is ethically problematic about NRP-cDCD is that the arteries providing blood flow to the brain are occluded to ensure that neurological function will not resume. The evident intentionality underlying this practice is to violate the DDR by bringing about the cessation of neurological function, which, I will argue

[13] An alternative version of this procedure provides circulation only to the abdominal organs, still occluding circulation to the brain.

[14] See https://www.uniformlaws.org/committees/community-home?CommunityKey=a1380d75-62bc-4a5b-ba3a-e74001a9ab57.

below, constitutes the true death of a human organism.[15] Again, this issue goes back to the original cDCD protocols:

> At the time that the individual is declared dead, it is quite possible that substantial portions of that person's brain (including the higher brain, responsible for thoughts and emotions) have not yet permanently ceased to function. If one, for example, were to restart pulmonary and cardiac function in that person, the brain (including the higher brain) might then be brought back to some degree of function (Menikoff 2002, p. 14).

> From a regulatory perspective, it is not necessary to establish that non-heart-beating donors would meet brain-based criteria for determining death … Nevertheless, from an ontological or metaphysical perspective, we can still ask whether it is possible for a person to be dead before his or her brain has died. Given the centrality of the role the brain plays in human life … it is difficult to see how a person with a living brain could be dead (DuBois 2002, pp. 34–35).

In its report, *Defining Death: Medical, Legal, and Ethical Issues in the Definition of Death*, the President's Commission (1981, pp. 34–37) affirmed two formulations of the whole-brain criterion. The first defines death as the irreversible cessation of an organism's "integrated functions" and contends that loss of cardiopulmonary function and loss of whole-brain function are equally suitable criteria for declaring death. The second recognizes the brain as the "primary organ" that is both "the sponsor of consciousness" and "the complex organizer and regulator of bodily functions." This view asserts that the loss of whole-brain function is the primary criterion for declaring death and affirms the loss of cardiopulmonary function as a practical surrogate. In what follows, I will defend the latter interpretation.

13.4 Brain Death as *True* Human Death

13.4.1 Defense of Brain Death[16]

Shewmon describes the brain as more a "regulator" or "fine-tuner" of the body's vital functions, rather than being constitutive of them, and thus integrative unity may persist in an adequately supported brain dead body. It does not seem, however, that this distinction makes a real difference in criticizing brain death. While brainstem functioning is certainly not solely responsible for the vital functions of circulation and respiration, a human body cannot carry out such functions on its own in the absence of brainstem functioning. The assumption of such functions by life-support machinery indicates that the body has lost the capacity to perform them under its own control. It thus remains arguable that integrative unity has been lost in such cases.

---

[15] For discussion of the evident intentionality underlying NRP-cDCD, see Karches and Eberl (2024). For broader ethical analyses of NRP-cDCD, see Karches et al. (2023) and Turner (2024).

[16] For a more complete defense of brain death and critique of Shewmon's arguments, see Eberl (2020, Ch. 6), from which this subsection is derived.

I contend that a human being remains biologically alive only if able to control one's vital functions such that they act in a *self-integrating* fashion and not in a merely *coordinated* fashion among themselves with no reference to their composing a larger, more complex organism. Maureen Condic (2016, p. 271) aptly explains this key distinction:

Integration: The compilation of information from diverse structures and systems to generate a response that (1) is multifaceted, (2) is context dependent, (3) takes into account the condition of the whole, and (4) regulates the activity of systems throughout the body for the sake of the continued health and function of the whole. Integration is (by definition) a global response and during postnatal stages of human life is uniquely accomplished by the nervous system, most especially the brain.

Coordination: The ability of a stimulus, acting through a specific signaling molecule, to bring responding cells into a common action or condition. Coordination can reflect either (1) a single type of response that occurs simultaneously in multiple cells or (2) a set of synchronous, but cell-type specific responses. Coordination can be local or global and is accomplished both by the brain and by other signaling systems.

In a brain dead body, there does persist a degree of *reactive functionality* of one organ or organ system in relation to another, which accounts for the fact that such a body may undergo the complex coordinated activities associated with, for example, physical maturation or fetal gestation; but it is a conceptual leap to describe such reactive functionality as "integration." Hence, the principled requirement that one must have the intrinsic capacity to *control* one's vital functions, which requires a functioning brain – particularly the brainstem – is a *sine qua non* for an organism to exist *as a living whole*. A key indication of the brain's essential role in somatic integration is its unique connection with every other part of the body:

> By contrast with other cells and organs that influence each other through molecular signalling locally and/or via the bloodstream, the brain is the *only* organ that can receive information *simultaneously* from *all* parts of the body, and can respond to that information by crafting a global, adaptive response that directs the functions of multiple bodily systems at once (Moschella 2017, pp. 754–755).

A human body without a functioning brain is like a "conductorless orchestra," each part playing its own role without any regard for the flourishing of the whole (Moschella 2019).

If one's brainstem is no longer intact and functional but a mechanical ventilator, ECMO, or cardiopulmonary bypass machine is utilized to support one's vital functions, then such functions and the capacity for performing them are no longer attributable to the individual. One would only passively receive the benefits – oxygenated air being introduced and circulated throughout one's body – that such support can provide.[17] Of course, other artificial mechanisms may also "take over" for vital functions of the body – for example, dialysis replacing kidney function or an insulin pump replacing pancreatic function – but these particular functions are not as central to a human organism's integrative unity as those which circulate oxygenated blood throughout the body, which is essential for all other organic functioning – in the absence of artificial replacement – to persist.

If, however, one's brainstem is intact and functional, then, regardless of whether one's dependence on artificial life-support is temporary – for example, a patient on cardiopulmonary bypass during an open-heart procedure – or permanent – such as an artificial heart or ventricular assist device – it does not follow that one no longer possesses integrative unity insofar as their functioning brainstem materially grounds their persistent capacity to actualize integrative control of their vital functions, even if other material conditions of one's body precludes ever actualizing such control.[18]

A human body loses integrative unity when it no longer has the intrinsic capacity to coordinate the vital functions of circulation and respiration – by virtue of an intact and functional brainstem – and such functions can be maintained only by artificial means. The clinical sign of this capacity being lost is the irreversible cessation of *spontaneous* heartbeat and respiration. These two vital functions are emphasized insofar as the circulation of oxygenated blood throughout the body is *the* fundamental biological requirement for any and all organic activity in the absence of technological replacement. While other functions – such as digestion, waste excretion, and immune response – are also *vital* for an organism to survive, the respective organs associated with these functions are dependent upon oxygenated blood being circulated through them.[19] It must be noted, however, that the functions of the kidneys and hormonal system are also required if oxygenated blood is to be circulated throughout the body. Nevertheless, such organic activity *supports*, but is not *constitutive* of, the vital activity that brings oxygen into the organic system (respiration) and transports it throughout the body (circulation). These other systems help *maintain* the transport system – i.e., blood – but do not effect the transport itself. Inductive support for this contention is the near-immediacy with which an organism dies with the cessation of circulatory/respiratory activity contrasted with the longer period required for an organism to perish due to renal or other systemic failures. Thus, the form of dependency a brain dead individual has with respect to a

[17] While the essential form of artificial life-support that precludes an individual having the capacity for vital functions is a mechanical ventilator, ECMO, or cardiopulmonary bypass machine, additional supportive treatment may need to be provided, such as the use of vasopressive drugs and other pharmaceuticals, to maintain the homeostatic conditions of body temperature, fluid and electrolyte balance, etc.

[18] For explication of the metaphysical import of the capacity/actualization distinction in this context, see Eberl (2008).

[19] The PCB (2008, pp. 62-64) also affirms the "indispensable" requirement of spontaneous breathing to assert, on their alternative biophilosophical foundation, that a human organism is "doing the work that constitutes – and preserves – it as a whole." They conclude, "The simulated 'breathing' that the ventilator makes possible is not, therefore, a *vital sign*: It is not a sign that the organism is accomplishing its vital work and thus remains a living whole."

mechanical ventilator or functionally similar device is quite different from that of a living human being who requires a pacemaker, insulin pump, or a similar device, to regulate or help maintain their vital functions.

Shewmon's claim that certain functions are "integrative" just because they are holistic does not follow.[20] Following Condic's distinction, such functions can be understood as emerging from the interaction of a body's organ systems in a coordinated fashion without entailing that they are integrated as a whole. I contend that a human body's having *control* over its vital functions of circulation and respiration is a necessary criterion for it to have integrative unity; these specific activities are *the* vital functions necessary for somatic integrative unity insofar as all other organs of the body depend upon oxygenated blood being circulated through them in order to survive and function. The case for abandoning brain death depends upon there being cases in which spontaneous heartbeat and respiration occur in the absence of whole-brain function, and such a case has not yet been presented.

13.4.2 Persistent Neuroendocrine Function

As noted above, the case of Jahi McMath and others who have experience long-term somatic survival – with supportive interventions such as mechanical ventilation, medically-provided nutrition and hydration, etc. – has ignited disagreement among brain death proponents regarding what biological functions constitute the necessary and sufficient conditions for determining the loss of integrative unity. Unquestionably, there must be irreversible loss of cerebral and brainstem function. But what about the hypothalamus, which Bernat's biophilosophical rationale supporting brain death specifically mentions as one of the brain's "critical functions"?

While the hypothalamus undoubtedly plays an important role in preserving a human organism's integrative unity by producing hormones related to reproduction and puberty, as well as telling the body to manage its fluid homeostasis, temperature, satiety, sleep, and blood pressure, it does not drive homeostatic function in the same way that, for example, the brainstem drives breathing. In the context of brain death – when the hypothalamus has lost its brain-mediated input/output connections – the only way for the hypothalamus to have any influence on the rest of the body is through the neuroendocrine pathways: hormonal secretion and regulation of

[20] In an exchange with Shewmon, Conrado Estol effectively demonstrates how such non-brain-mediated functions fail to qualify as "holistic," while José Masdeu challenges Shewmon's contention by comparing the presence of the properties he lists in both a whole-brain dead body and an artificially maintained hand (Sorondo 2007, pp. xxxv–xxxvii). David Hershenov points out that corpses also possess properties, such as bloating and rigor mortis, which are both *emergent* – that is, they are not properties of the parts – and *holistic* – that is, they apply to the body as a whole (personal correspondence).

osmotic homeostasis through the secretion of the hormone vasopressin.[21] Does such neuroendocrine function alone constitute the integrated functioning of an "organism as a whole"?

Unfortunately, no additional biological data can help answer this question, as it is subject to interpretation within a particular biophilosophical framework. It is worth noting, though, that the hypothalamus connects to various organ systems beyond the central nervous system. Some commentators have emphasized the hypothalamic connection to the reproductive system, noting the onset of puberty in the cases of McMath, T.K., and others as ontologically significant (Sulmasy et al. 2024; Sulmasy and DeCock 2023). But why privilege the reproductive system above other systems to which the hypothalamus is functionally connected? Would persistent functioning of the integumentary system (hair, skin and nails) suffice for someone to be alive? If we do not require loss of function of all organ systems for an organism to cease existing as an integrated whole, why cannot loss of central nervous system function be the sole necessary and sufficient condition for declaring death? Further, many animals – and even some humans[22] – go through life without experiencing puberty; but no human can live without circulating oxygenated blood.

Indeed, people can live well without a hypothalamus – e.g., after removal from surgery due to a tumor extraction – with exogenous hormonal replacement. The brain's other structures can be irreversibly destroyed – with no potential for recovery – and the hypothalamus can be preserved because of collateral blood flow from vessels external to the brain if organ support is maintained via intravenous fluids and a ventilator to stabilize blood pressure and oxygen levels. Thus, while it is the case *anatomically* with hypothalamic function preserved that not all functions of the entire brain have ceased, it is the case *functionally* that patients determined to be dead by neurological criteria "will never regain consciousness or breathe independently again, irrespective of whether neuroendocrine function is present or not" (Thomas and Manara 2022, p. 123).

We thus return to the role of the hypothalamus with respect to the integrative unity of a living human body. Does the hypothalamus fulfill a "critical function" in terms of bodily integration, control, or behavior? For the reasons outlined above, it is evident it does not. While playing an important role, there is no evidence that hypothalamic function is either necessary or sufficient for the persistent integrative life of a mature human organism. In fact, it is not substantively different from the function of other endocrine glands like the adrenal glands that lie above the kidneys, yet no one believes testing for adrenal function is relevant for determining death. It is a mistake to assert the hypothalamus's location as being more relevant than its function. This is why some other legal jurisdictions, such as the UK, require only irreversible cessation of brainstem function, given its unique and irreplaceable role

[21] I am grateful for E. Wesley Ely and Allen Aksamit for helpful input on the relevant neurobiological considerations here.

[22] For example, those with Kallmann Syndrome: https://medlineplus.gov/genetics/condition/kallmann-syndrome/.

in preserving and regulating cardiopulmonary function (Pallis 1982).[23] Therefore, I conclude that the hypothalamus, while performing critical regulatory functions, is not a *sine qua non* with respect to the human body's integrative unity. Rather, the spontaneous and self-regulated circulation of oxygenated blood, accomplished by the heart and lungs through the mediation of the brainstem, is that without which a human body cannot sustain itself as a living organism.

If brain death constitutes the true death of a human being, then the circulatory criterion may function as a surrogate indicator assuming a sufficient waiting period is allowed before organ procurement begins, which would be problematic for DCD protocols, including NRP-cDCD. As Jerry Menikoff (1998, p. 160) notes,

> It would indeed be disingenuous to claim that X [loss of cardiopulmonary function] is being used as a surrogate for Y [loss of whole-brain function] while interpreting the statute [UDDA] to allow reliance on X at a time when one is certain that Y has not yet occurred.

Menikoff (1998, p. 158) further asserts, "Irreversibility is a statement about the physical state of our world and our *ability* to alter it," not a statement about what we *elect* to alter. In short, we should not "mistake the 'prognosis of death' for the 'diagnosis' of death'" (Zamperetti et al. 2003, p. 183).

13.5 Conclusion

As Aristotle (2019, bk. 1, ch. 3) noted, moral science can only provide the degree of certainty its subject matter allows; hence, we cannot expect the same degree of certainty in our moral reasoning as we can in other areas of inquiry, such as logic or mathematics. We must thus reason toward *moral certitude*; in other words, we must aim toward as much certainty as can be reasonably had that we are acting morally (Haas 2008). But what are the criteria for claiming moral certitude in ethical matters such as when we can procure vital organs from putatively dead human beings? In the face of reasonable doubt, should we err on the side of caution and not risk causing death because we have utilized the wrong criterion? (Brugger 2016) Or, should we balance such risk with the potential benefits to those whose lives may be prolonged through organ transplantation? Two opposing responses, neither of which I endorse, are either to await the onset of putrefaction as the sure sign that death has occurred (Oderberg 2019), precluding any possibility of organ transplantation, or, in order to respect autonomy and diverse cultural and religious perspectives, to abandon the DDR and allow individuals or their families to decide for themselves which criterion of death – even including higher-brain death – ought to be employed in each case (Miller and Truog 2011; Veatch 1993).

---

[23] Note that I am not advocating for a solely brainstem-based criterion of death as it does not rule out persistent neocortical function, which I contend is essential for a human being's death (Eberl 2005).

While it is certainly the case that clinical criteria and diagnostic tests for determining brain death ought to be continually revisited and critiqued – as well as ensuring uniform compliance with such criteria[24] – the biophilosophical validity of brain death remains justified. The use of the whole-brain criterion not only respects the DDR in organ procurement, but also allows for families of brain dead individuals to cease resuscitative or life-sustaining interventions that only serve to generate false hope of recovery.[25]

References

Ad Hoc Committee of the Harvard Medical School. 1968. A Definition of Irreversible Coma. *Journal of the American Medical Association* 205 (6): 337–340.

American College of Physicians [ACP]. 2021. *Ethics, Determination of Death, and Organ Transplantation in Normothermic Regional Perfusion (NRP) with Controlled Donation After Circulatory Determination of Death (cDCD): American College of Physicians Statement of Concern.* April 17: https://www.acponline.org/acp_policy/policies/ethics_determination_of_death_and_organ_transplantation_in_nrp_2021.pdf.

Aristotle. 2019. *Nicomachean Ethics, trans. Terence Irwin.* 3rd ed. Indianapolis: Hackett.

Austriaco, Nicanor. 2003. Is the Brain-Dead Patient *Really* Dead? *Studia Moralia* 41 (2): 277–308.

Aviv, Rachel. 2018. What Does It Mean to Die? *The New Yorker*, January 29: https://www.newyorker.com/magazine/2018/02/05/what-does-it-mean-to-die.

Bernat, James L. 1998. A Defense of the Whole-Brain Concept of Death. *Hastings Center Report* 28 (2): 14–23.

Bernat, James L. 1999. Refinements in the Definition and Criterion of Death. In *The Definition of Death: Contemporary Controversies*, ed. S. Youngner, R. Arnold, and R. Shapiro, 83–92. Baltimore: Johns Hopkins University Press.

Bernat, James L. 2001. Philosophical and Ethical Aspects of Brain Death. In *Brain Death*, ed. Eelco F. M. Wijdicks. Philadelphia: Lippincott, Williams, and Wilkins.

Bernat, James L. 2002. The Biophilosophical Basis of Whole-Brain Death. *Social Philosophy and Policy* 19:324–342.

Bernat, James L. 2008a. Terri Schiavo's Tragedy and Ours Too. *Neurology* 71 (13): 964–965.

Bernat, James L. 2008b. *Ethical Issues in Neurology.* 3rd ed. Philadelphia: Lippincott, Williams, and Wilkins.

Bernat, James L. 2019. Refinements in the Organism as a Whole Rationale for Brain Death. *Linacre Quarterly* 86 (4): 347–358.

Bernat, James L. 2024. The Unified Brain-Based Determination of Death Conceptually Justifies Death Determination in DCDD and NRP Protocols. *American Journal of Bioethics* 24 (6): 4–15.

Bernat, James L., M. Culver, and B. Gert. 1981. On the Definition and Criterion of Death. *Annals of Internal Medicine* 94:389–394.

Bernstein, I., M. Watson, G. Simons, P. Catalano, G. Davis, and R. Collins. 1989. Maternal Brain Death and Prolonged Fetal Survival. *Obstetrics and Gynecology* 74:434–437.

[24] For studies of widespread variability in adherence to AAN guidelines for brain death determination, see Greer et al. (2016), Junn and Hwang (2019), and Dalle and Bernat (2020).

[25] It is important to note that the issue of establishing morally appropriate criteria to determine death extends well beyond organ donation since about only two percent of all in-hospital deaths are declared using neurological criteria and only about twenty percent of the patients declared brain dead become organ donors (Seifi et al. 2020; Qu et al. 2021).

Bonelli, J., E. H. Prat, N. Auner, and R. Bonelli. 1999. Brain Death: Understanding the Organism as a Whole. *Medicina e Morale* 3:497–515.

Brugger, E. Christian. 2016. Are Brain Dead Individuals Dead? Grounds for Reasonable Doubt. *Journal of Medicine and Philosophy* 41 (3): 329–350.

Busch, Emil J. N. 2024. Restoring the Organism as a Whole: Does NRP Resurrect the Dead? *American Journal of Bioethics* 24 (6): 27–33.

Caplan, Arthur L. 2014. Little Girl Is Brain Dead: Don't Give Family False Hope. *Medscape*. January 22: https://www.medscape.com/viewarticle/819307?form=fpf.

Condic, Maureen L. 2016. Determination of Death: A Scientific Perspective on Biological Integration. *Journal of Medicine and Philosophy* 41 (3): 257–278.

Dalle, Anne L., and James L. Bernat. 2020. Inconsistencies Between the Criterion and Tests for Brain Death. *Journal of Intensive Care Medicine* 35 (8): 772–780.

Dillon, W. P., R. V. Lee, M. J. Tronolone, S. Buckwald, and R. J. Foote. 1982. Life Support and Maternal Brain Death during Pregnancy. *JAMA* 248:1089–1091.

DuBois, James M. 1999. Non-Heart-Beating Organ Donation: A Defense of the Required Determination of Death. *Journal of Law, Medicine, and Ethics* 27:126–136.

DuBois, James M. 2002. Is Organ Procurement Causing the Death of Patients? *Issues in Law and Medicine* 18:21–41.

Eberl, Jason T. 2005. A Thomistic Understanding of Human Death. *Bioethics* 19 (1): 29–48.

Eberl, Jason T. 2008. Potentiality, Possibility, and the Irreversibility of Death. *Review of Metaphysics* 62 (1): 61–77.

Eberl, Jason T. 2020. *The Nature of Human Persons: Metaphysics and Bioethics*. Notre Dame: University of Notre Dame Press.

Field, D. R., E. A. Gates, R. K. Creasy, A. R. Jonsen, and R. K. Laros. 1988. Maternal Brain Death During Pregnancy: Medical and Ethical Issues. *JAMA* 260:816–822.

Greer, David M., Hilary H. Wang, Jennifer D. Robinson, Panayiotis N. Varelas, Galen V. Henderson, and Eelco F. M. Wijdicks. 2016. Variability of Brain Death Policies in the United States. *JAMA Neurology* 73 (2): 213–218.

Greer, David M., Matthew P. Kirschen, Ariane Lewis, Gary S. Gronseth, Alexander Rae-Grant, Stephen Ashwal, Maya A. Babu, David F. Bauer, Lori Billinghurst, Amanda Corey, Sonia Partap, Michael A. Rubin, Lori Shutter, Courtney Takahashi, Robert C. Tasker, Panayiotis Nicolaou Varelas, Eelco Wijdicks, Amy Bennett, Scott R. Wessels, and John J. Halperin. 2023. Pediatric and Adult Brain Death/Death by Neurologic Criteria Consensus Guideline. *Neurology* 101 (24): 1112–1132.

Haas, John M. 2008. Absolute Versus Prudential Certitude in Criteria for Determining Death. *Ethics and Medics* 33 (7):

Institute of Medicine. 1997. *Non-Heart-Beating Organ Transplantation: Medical and Ethical Issues in Procurement*. Washington, D.C.: National Academy Press.

Institute of Medicine. 2000. *Non-Heart-Beating Organ Transplantation: Practice and Protocols*. Washington, D.C.: National Academy Press.

Johnson, L. S. M. 2016. The Case for Reasonable Accommodation of Conscientious Objections to Declarations of Brain Death. *Journal of Bioethical Inquiry* 13 (1): 105–115.

Jonsen, Albert R. 1998. *The Birth of Bioethics*. New York: Oxford University Press.

Junn, Alexandra, and David Y. Hwang. 2019. Practice Variability in Determination of Death by Neurologic Criteria for Adult Patients. *Yale Journal of Biology and Medicine* 92 (4): 719–724.

Karakatsanis, K. G., and J. N. Tsanakas. 2002. A Critique of the Concept of 'Brain Death'. *Issues in Law and Medicine* 18:127–141.

Karches, Kyle E., and Jason T. Eberl. 2024. Distinguishing Ethical from Diagnostic Concerns About NRP-cDCD. *American Journal of Bioethics* 24 (6): 68–71.

Karches, Kyle E., Erica K. Salter, and Patrick McCruden. 2023. Dead Enough? NRP-cDCD and Remaining Questions for the Ethics of DCD Protocols. *American Journal of Bioethics* 23 (2): 41–43.

Lewis, Ariane, Richard J. Bonnie, Thaddeus Pope, Leon G. Epstein, David M. Greer, Matthew P. Kirschen, Michael Rubin, and James A. Russell. 2019. Determination of Death by Neurologic Criteria in the United States: The Case for Revising the Uniform Determination of Death Act. *Journal of Law, Medicine, and Ethics* 47 (4): 9–24.

Lewis, Ariane, Richard J. Bonnie, and Thaddeus Pope. 2020. It's Time to Revise the Uniform Determination of Death Act. *Annals of Internal Medicine* 172 (2): 143–144.

Lizza, John P. 2006. *Persons, Humanity, and the Definition of Death.* Baltimore: Johns Hopkins University Press.

Menikoff, Jerry. 1998. Doubts About Death: The Silence of the Institute of Medicine. *Journal of Law, Medicine and Ethics* 26: 157–165.

Menikoff, Jerry. 2002. The Importance of Being Dead: Non-Heart-Beating Organ Donation. *Issues in Law and Medicine* 18: 3–20.

Miller, Franklin G., and Robert D. Truog. 2011. *Death, Dying, and Organ Transplantation: Reconstructing Medical Ethics at the End of Life.* New York: Oxford University Press.

Moschella, Melissa. 2017. Complexity of Defining Death: Organismal Death Does Not Mean the Cessation of All Biological Life. *Journal of Medical Ethics* 43 (11): 754–755.

Moschella, Melissa. 2019. The Human Organism Is Not a Conductorless Orchestra: A Defense of Brain Death as True Biological Death. *Theoretical Medicine and Bioethics* 40 (5): 437–453.

Nair-Collins, Michael. 2023. Must Hypothalamic Neurosecretory Function Cease for Brain Death Determination? Yes: The UDDA Revision Series. *Neurology* 101 (3): 134–136.

Nair-Collins, Michael, and Ari R. Joffe. 2023. Frequent Preservation of Neurologic Function in Brain Death and Brainstem Death Entails False-Positive Misdiagnosis and Cerebral Perfusion. *AJOB Neuroscience* 14 (3): 255–268.

Nair-Collins, Michael, and F. G. Miller. 2017. Do the 'Brain Dead' Merely Appear to Be Alive? *Journal of Medical Ethics* 43:747–753.

Nair-Collins, Michael, Jesse Northrup, and James Olcese. 2016. Hypothalamic–Pituitary Function in Brain Death: A Review. *Journal of Intensive Care Medicine* 31 (1): 41–50.

Oderberg, David S. 2019. Death, Unity, and the Brain. *Theoretical Medicine and Bioethics* 40 (5): 359–379.

Olick, Robert S. 1991. Brain Death, Religious Freedom, and Public Policy: New Jersey's Landmark Legislative Initiative. *Kennedy Institute of Ethics Journal* 1 (4): 275–288.

Omelianchuk, Adam. 2021. Brain Death as the End of a Human Organism as a Self-Moving Whole. *Journal of Medicine and Philosophy* 46:530–560.

Pallis, Christopher. 1982. ABC of Brain Stem Death: From Brain Death to Brain Stem Death. *British Medical Journal* 285:1487–1490.

Parent, B., A. Caplan, N. Moazami, and R. Montgomery. 2022. Response to American College of Physician's Statement on the Ethics of Transplant After Normothermic Regional Perfusion. *American Journal of Transplantation* 22 (5): 1307–1310.

Potts, Michael, Paul A. Byrne, and Richard G. Nilges, eds. 2000. *Beyond Brain Death: The Case Against Brain Based Criteria for Human Death.* Dordrecht: Springer.

President's Commission for the Study of Ethical Problems in Medicine and Biomedical and Behavioral Research. 1981. *Defining Death: Medical, Legal and Ethical Issues in the Determination of Death.* Washington, D.C.: U.S. Government Printing Office.

President's Council on Bioethics [PCB]. 2008. *Controversies in the Determination of Death.* Washington, D.C.: President's Council on Bioethics.

Qu, Zhi, Carina Oedingen, Tim Bartling, Jan Beneke, Michael Zink, Christian Krauth, and Harald Schrem. 2021. Systematic Review on Potential Brain Dead Donor Estimations and Conversion Rates to Actually Realized Organ Donations. *Transplantation Reviews* 35 (4): 100638.

Repertinger, Susan, William P. Fitzgibbons, Matthew F. Omojola, and Roger A. Brumback. 2006. Long Survival Following Bacterial Meningitis-Associated Brain Destruction. *Journal of Child Neurology* 21:591–595.

Robbins, Nathaniel M., and James L. Bernat. 2020. What Should We Do About the Mismatch Between Legal Criteria for Death and How Brain Death Is Diagnosed? *AMA Journal of Ethics*.

December: https://journalofethics.ama-assn.org/article/what-should-we-do-about-mismatch-between-legal-criteria-death-and-how-brain-death-diagnosed/2020-12.

Robertson, J. A. 2000. The Dead Donor Rule. *Hastings Center Report* 29:6–14.

Scherz, Paul. 2022. How the Body Became Integrated: Cybernetics in the History of the Brain Death Debate. *Journal of Medicine and Philosophy* 47 (3): 387–406.

Seifi, Ali, John Vincent Lacci, and Daniel Agustin Godoy. 2020. Incidence of Brain Death in the United States. *Clinical Neurology and Neurosurgery* 195:105885.

Shewmon, D. Alan. 1985. The Metaphysics of Brain Death, Persistent Vegetative State, and Dementia. *The Thomist* 49:24–80.

Shewmon, D. Alan. 1992. 'Brain Death': A Valid Theme with Invalid Variations, Blurred by Semantic Ambiguity. In *Working Group on the Determination of Brain Death and Its Relationship to Human Death*, ed. R. J. White, H. Angstwurm, and I. Carrasco de Paula, 23–51. Pontifical Academy of Sciences: Vatican City.

Shewmon, D. Alan. 1997. Recovery from 'Brain Death': A Neurologist's *Apologia*. *Linacre Quarterly* 64 (1): 30–96.

Shewmon, D. Alan. 1998a. 'Brainstem Death,' 'Brain Death' and Death: A Critical Re-Evaluation of the Purported Equivalence. *Issues in Law and Medicine* 14:125–145.

Shewmon, D. Alan. 1998b. Chronic 'Brain Death': Meta-Analysis and Conceptual Consequences. *Neurology* 51:1538–1545.

Shewmon, D. Alan. 2001. The Brain and Somatic Integration: Insights into the Standard Biological Rationale for Equating 'Brain Death' with Death. *Journal of Medicine and Philosophy* 26:457–478.

Shewmon, D. Alan. 2004. The 'Critical Organ' for the Organism as a Whole: Lessons from the Lowly Spinal Cord. In *Brain Death and Disorders of Consciousness*, ed. Calixto Machado and D. Alan Shewmon. Dordrecht: Springer.

Shewmon, D. Alan. 2007. Mental Disconnect: 'Physiological Decapitation' as a Heuristic for Understanding 'Brain Death'. In *Working Group on the Signs of Death*, ed. Marcelo Sánchez Sorondo, 292–333. Vatican City: Pontifical Academy of Sciences.

Shewmon, D. Alan. 2009. Brain Death: Can It Be Resuscitated? *Hastings Center Report* 39 (2): 18–24.

Shewmon, D. Alan. 2018. Truly Reconciling the Case of Jahi McMath. *Neurocritical Care* 29:165–170.

Shewmon, D. Alan, and Noriko Salamon. 2021. The Extraordinary Case of Jahi McMath. *Perspectives in Biology and Medicine* 64 (4): 457–478.

Sorondo, M. S. 2007. *The Signs of Death*. Vatican City: Pontifical Academy of Sciences.

Stevens, Robert. 2014. The Ethics Of Being Brain Dead: Doctors and Bioethicists Discuss Jahi McMath And Marlise Munoz. *Huffpost*. January 10: https://www.huffpost.com/entry/ethics-brain-dead_n_4577116.

Sulmasy, Daniel P. 2019. Whole-Brain Death and Integration: Realigning the Ontological Concept with Clinical Diagnostic Tests. *Theoretical Medicine and Bioethics* 40:455–481.

Sulmasy, Daniel P., and Christopher A. DeCock. 2023. Rethinking Brain Death—Why 'Dead Enough' Is Not Good Enough. *Neurology* 101:320–325.

Sulmasy, Daniel P., Christopher A. DeCock, Carlo S. Tornatore, Allen H. Roberts II, James Giordano, and G. Kevin Donovan. 2024. A Biophilosophical Approach to the Determination of Brain Death. *CHEST* 165 (4): 959–966.

Thomas, Ian, and Alex R. Manara. 2022. Preserved Hypothalamic Function Does Not Preclude Determination of Death by Neurologic Criteria. In *Death Determination by Neurologic Criteria: Areas of Consensus and Controversy*, ed. Ariane Lewis and James L. Bernat, 117–127. Dordrecht: Springer.

Turner, Barrett. 2024. Thoraco-abdominal Normothermic Regional Perfusion (TA-NRP) Resuscitates Moral Doubts about Donation after Circulatory Death (DCD). *Health Care Ethics USA* 32 (1): 33–39.

Veatch, Robert M. 1993. The Impending Collapse of the Whole-Brain Definition of Death. *Hastings Center Report* 23 (4): 18–24.

Veatch, Robert M., and Lainie F. Ross. 2016. *Defining Death: The Case for Choice*. Washington, D.C.: Georgetown University Press.

Zamperetti, N., R. Bellomo, and C. Ronco. 2003. Defining Death in Non-Heart Beating Organ Donors. *Journal of Medical Ethics* 29:182–185.

Zaner, Richard M., ed. 1988. *Death: Beyond Whole-Brain Criteria*. Dordrecht: Springer.

Appendix

L. M. Rasmussen, S. Holm (eds.), *50 Years of Philosophy and Medicine*, Philosophy and Medicine 150, https://doi.org/10.1007/978-3-031-95175-6

Volume_ number	Publication date	Short_title	Author editor 1	Author editor 2	Author editor 3	ISBN
1	1975-03-31	Engelhardt Jr. (Eds), Evaluation and Explanation in the Biomedical Sciences (Philosophy and Medicine 1)	H. Tristram Engelhardt Jr.	S.F. Spicker		978-90-277-0553-2
2	1976-03-31	Spicker (Eds), Philosophical Dimensions of the Neuro-Medical Sciences (Philosophy and Medicine 2)	S.F. Spicker	H. Tristram Engelhardt Jr.		978-90-277-0672-0
3	1977-08-31	Spicker (Eds), Philosophical Medical Ethics: Its Nature and Significance (Philosophy and Medicine 3)	S.F. Spicker	H. Tristram Engelhardt Jr.		978-90-277-0772-7
4	1977-12-31	Engelhardt Jr. (Eds), Mental Health: Philosophical Perspectives (Philosophy and Medicine 4)	H. Tristram Engelhardt Jr.	S.F. Spicker		978-90-277-0828-1
5	1980-07-31	Brody (Eds), Mental Illness: Law and Public Policy (Philosophy and Medicine 5)	B.A. Brody	H. Tristram Engelhardt Jr.		978-90-277-1057-4
6	1979-07-31	Engelhardt Jr. (Eds), Clinical Judgment: A Critical Appraisal (Philosophy and Medicine 6)	H. Tristram Engelhardt Jr.	S.F. Spicker	B. Towers	978-90-277-0952-3
7	1978-04-30	Spicker (Ed), Organism, Medicine, and Metaphysics (Philosophy and Medicine 7)	S.F. Spicker			978-90-277-0823-6
8	1981-01-31	Shelp (Ed), Justice and Health Care (Philosophy and Medicine 8)	E.E. Shelp			978-90-277-1251-6
9	1981-04-30	Spicker (Eds), The Law-Medicine Relation: A Philosophical Exploration (Philosophy and Medicine 9)	S.F. Spicker	Y.M. Healey Jr.	H. Tristram Engelhardt Jr.	978-90-277-1217-2
10	1982-01-31	Bondeson (Eds), New Knowledge in the Biomedical Sciences (Philosophy and Medicine 10)	W.B. Bondeson	H. Tristram Engelhardt Jr.	S.F. Spicker	978-90-277-1319-3
11	1982-05-31	Shelp (Ed), Beneficence and Health Care (Philosophy and Medicine 11)	E.E. Shelp			978-90-277-1377-3
12	1982-10-31	Agich, Responsibility in Health Care (Philosophy and Medicine 12)	G.J. Agich			978-90-277-1417-6
13	1983-06-30	Bondeson (Eds), Abortion and the Status of the Fetus (Philosophy and Medicine 13)	W.B. Bondeson	H. Tristram Engelhardt Jr.	S.F. Spicker	978-90-277-1493-0
14	1983-09-30	Shelp (Ed), The Clinical Encounter (Philosophy and Medicine 14)	E.E. Shelp			978-90-277-1593-7

15	1984-02-29	Moskop (Eds), Ethics and Mental Retardation (Philosophy and Medicine 15)	J.C. Moskop	L.M. Kopelman		978-90-277-1630-9
16	1984-05-31	Nordenfelt (Eds), Health, Disease, and Causal Explanations in Medicine (Philosophy and Medicine 16)	L.Y Nordenfelt	B.I.B Lindahl		978-90-277-1660-6
17	1985-03-31	Shelp (Ed), Virtue and Medicine (Philosophy and Medicine 17)	E.E. Shelp			978-90-277-1808-2
18	1985-03-31	Carrick, Medical Ethics in Antiquity (Philosophy and Medicine 18)	P. Carrick			978-90-277-1825-9
19	1985-09-30	Moskop (Eds), Ethics and Critical Care Medicine (Philosophy and Medicine 19)	J.C. Moskop	L.M. Kopelman		978-90-277-1820-4
20	1985-09-30	Shelp (Ed), Theology and Bioethics (Philosophy and Medicine 20)	E.E. Shelp			978-90-277-1857-0
21	1986-11-30	Agich (Eds), The Price of Health (Philosophy and Medicine 21)	G.J. Agich	C.E. Begley		978-90-277-2285-0
22	1986-11-30	Shelp (Ed), Sexuality and Medicine (Philosophy and Medicine 22)	E.E. Shelp			978-90-277-2290-4
23	1987-03-31	Shelp (Ed), Sexuality and Medicine (Philosophy and Medicine 23)	E.E. Shelp			978-1-55608-013-5
24	1987-03-31	McMillan (Eds), Euthanasia and the Newborn (Philosophy and Medicine 24)	R.C. McMillan	H. Tristram Engelhardt Jr.	S.F. Spicker	978-90-277-2299-7
25	1987-10-31	Spicker (Eds), Ethical Dimensions of Geriatric Care (Philosophy and Medicine 25)	S.F. Spicker	S.R. Ingman	Ian Lawson	978-1-55608-027-2
26	1987-09-30	Nordenfelt, On the Nature of Health (Philosophy and Medicine 26)	L.Y Nordenfelt			978-1-55608-032-6
27	1987-10-31	Spicker (Eds), The Contraceptive Ethos (Philosophy and Medicine 27)	S.F. Spicker	W.B. Bondeson	H. Tristram Engelhardt Jr.	978-1-55608-035-7
28	1988-05-31	Spicker (Eds), The Use of Human Beings in Research (Philosophy and Medicine 28)	S.F. Spicker	I. Alon	A. de Vries	978-1-55608-043-2

(continued)

Volume_ number	Publication date	Short_title	Author editor 1	Author editor 2	Author editor 3	ISBN
29	1988-04-30	King (Eds), The Physician as Captain of the Ship (Philosophy and Medicine 29)	N.M. King	L.R. Churchill	Alan W. Cross	978-1-55608-044-9
30	1988-09-30	Sass (Eds), Health Care Systems (Philosophy and Medicine 30)	Hans-Martin Sass	R.U. Massey		978-1-55608-045-6
31	1988-05-31	Zaner (Ed), Death: Beyond Whole-Brain Criteria (Philosophy and Medicine 31)	Richard M. Zaner			978-1-55608-053-1
32	1988-09-30	Brody (Ed), Moral Theory and Moral Judgments in Medical Ethics (Philosophy and Medicine 32)	B.A. Brody			978-1-55608-060-9
33	1989-02-28	Kopelman (Eds), Children and Health Care (Philosophy and Medicine 33)	L.M. Kopelman	J.C. Moskop		978-1-55608-078-4
34	1989-03-31	Pellegrino (Eds), Catholic Perspectives on Medical Morals (Philosophy and Medicine 34)	Edmund D. Pellegrino	J. Langan	John Collins Harvey	978-1-55608-083-8
35	1989-08-31	Brody (Ed), Suicide and Euthanasia (Philosophy and Medicine 35)	B.A. Brody			978-0-7923-0106-6
36	1990-08-31	Ten Have (Eds), The Growth of Medical Knowledge (Philosophy and Medicine 36)	H.A. Ten Have	G.L Kimsma	S.F. Spicker	978-0-7923-0736-5
37	1990-10-31	Löwy (Ed), The Polish School of Philosophy of Medicine (Philosophy and Medicine 37)	Ilana Löwy			978-0-7923-0958-1
38	1991-07-31	Bole III/Bondeson, Rights to Health Care (Philosophy and Medicine 38)	Thomas J. Bole III	W.B. Bondeson		978-0-7923-1137-9
39	1991-10-31	Gardell Cutter (Eds), Competency (Philosophy and Medicine 39)	Mary Ann Gardell Cutter	E.E. Shelp		978-0-7923-1304-5
40	1992-06-30	Peset (Eds), The Ethics of Diagnosis (Philosophy and Medicine 40)	José Luis Peset	Diego Gracia Guillén		978-0-7923-1544-5
42	1992-05-31	Toombs, The Meaning of Illness (Philosophy and Medicine 42)	S. Kay Toombs			978-0-7923-1570-4
43	1992-08-31	Leder (Ed), The Body in Medical Thought and Practice (Philosophy and Medicine 43)	D. Leder			978-0-7923-1657-2

44	1993-04-30	Delkeskamp-Hayes (Eds), Science, Technology, and the Art of Medicine (Philosophy and Medicine 44)	C. Delkeskamp-Hayes	Mary Ann Gardell Cutter		978-0-7923-1869-9
45	1993-03-31	Baker (Eds), The Codification of Medical Morality (Philosophy and Medicine 45)	R.B. Baker		R. Porter	978-0-7923-1921-4
46	1994-05-31	Bayertz (Ed), The Concept of Moral Consensus (Philosophy and Medicine 46)	K. Bayertz			978-0-7923-2615-1
48	1995-04-30	Baker (Eds), Legislating Medical Ethics (Philosophy and Medicine 48)	R.B. Baker	M. Strosberg		978-0-7923-2995-4
49	1995-10-31	Baker (Ed), The Codification of Medical Morality (Philosophy and Medicine 49)	R.B. Baker			978-0-7923-3529-0
50	1997-08-31	Carson (Eds), Philosophy of Medicine and Bioethics (Philosophy and Medicine 50)	Ronald A. Carson	C.R. Burns		978-0-7923-3545-0
51	1995-10-31	Wildes (Ed), Critical Choices and Critical Care (Philosophy and Medicine 51)	Kevin Wm. Wildes			978-0-7923-3701-0
52	1996-04-30	Bayertz (Ed), Sanctity of Life and Human Dignity (Philosophy and Medicine 52)	K. Bayertz			978-0-7923-3739-3
54	1996-11-30	Hoshino (Ed), Japanese and Western Bioethics (Philosophy and Medicine 54)	K. Hoshino			978-0-7923-4112-3
55	1997-12-31	Agius (Eds), Germ-Line Intervention and Our Responsibilities to Future Generations (Philosophy and Medicine 55)	Emmanuel Agius	S. Busuttil		978-0-7923-4828-3
56	1998-04-30	McCullough, John Gregory and the Invention of Professional Medical Ethics and the Profession of Medicine (Philosophy and Medicine 56)	Laurence B. McCullough			978-0-7923-4917-4
60	1999-06-30	Cherry (Ed), Persons and Their Bodies: Rights, Responsibilities, Relationships (Philosophy and Medicine 60)	Mark J. Cherry			978-0-7923-5701-8

(continued)

Volume_ number	Publication date	Short_title	Author editor 1	Author editor 2	Author editor 3	ISBN
62	1999-11-30	Kopelman (Ed), Building Bioethics (Philosophy and Medicine 62)	L.M. Kopelman			978-0-7923-5853-4
63	1999-11-30	Stempsey, Disease and Diagnosis (Philosophy and Medicine 63)	William E. Stempsey			978-0-7923-6029-2
64	2000-07-31	Engelhardt Jr. (Ed), The Philosophy of Medicine (Philosophy and Medicine 64)	H. Tristram Engelhardt Jr.			978-0-7923-6223-4
65	2000-06-30	Wear (Eds), Ethical Issues in Health Care on the Frontiers of the Twenty-First Century (Philosophy and Medicine 65)	S. Wear	J.J. Bono	G. Logue	978-0-7923-6277-7
66	2000-09-30	Potts (Eds), Beyond Brain Death (Philosophy and Medicine 66)	M. Potts	P.A. Byrne	R.G. Nilges	978-0-7923-6578-5
67	2001-10-31	Kopelman (Eds), Physician-Assisted Suicide: What are the Issues? (Philosophy and Medicine 67)	L.M. Kopelman	K.A. de Ville		978-0-7923-7142-7
68	2001-12-31	Toombs (Ed), Handbook of Phenomenology and Medicine (Philosophy and Medicine 68)	S. Kay Toombs			978-1-4020-0200-7
69	2001-12-31	Arts (Eds), Solidarity in Health and Social Care in Europe (Philosophy and Medicine 69)	R. ter Meulen	R. Muffels		978-1-4020-0164-2
70	2001-12-31	Nordgren, Responsible Genetics (Philosophy and Medicine 70)	A. Nordgren			978-1-4020-0201-4
72	2002-05-31	Taboada (Eds), Person, Society and Value (Philosophy and Medicine 72)	Paulina Taboada	K.F. Cuddeback	P. Donohue-White	978-1-4020-0503-9
73	2002-04-30	Li, Can Death Be a Harm to the Person Who Dies? (Philosophy and Medicine 73)	J. Li			978-1-4020-0505-3
75	2002-12-31	Parker (Eds), Mutating Concepts, Evolving Disciplines: Genetics, Medicine, and Society (Philosophy and Medicine 75)	L.S. Parker	Rachel A. Ankeny		978-1-4020-1040-8
76	2002-12-31	Bondeson (Eds), The Ethics of Managed Care: Professional Integrity and Patient Rights (Philosophy and Medicine 76)	W.B. Bondeson	J.W. Jones		978-1-4020-1045-3

77	2002-12-31	Vaux (Eds), Covenants of Life (Philosophy and Medicine 77)	K.L. Vaux	M. Stenberg		978-1-4020-1053-8
78	2004-03-31	Khushf (Ed), Handbook of Bioethics: (Philosophy and Medicine 78)	G. Khushf			978-1-4020-1870-1
79	2003-12-31	Smith Iltis (Ed), Institutional Integrity in Health Care (Philosophy and Medicine 79)	Ana Smith Iltis			978-1-4020-1782-7
81	2003-12-31	Gardell Cutter, Reframing Disease Contextually (Philosophy and Medicine 81)	Mary Ann Gardell Cutter			978-1-4020-1796-4
82	2004-10-29	Seifert, The Philosophical Diseases of Medicine and their Cure (Philosophy and Medicine 82)	Josef Seifert			978-1-4020-2870-0
86	2005-04-22	Cooper, Classifying Madness (Philosophy and Medicine 86)	Rachel Cooper			978-1-4020-3344-5
87	2005-09-13	Rasmussen (Ed), Ethics Expertise (Philosophy and Medicine 87)	Lisa Rasmussen			978-1-4020-3819-8
88	2006-05-04	Rawlinson (Eds), The Voice of Breast Cancer in Medicine and Bioethics (Philosophy and Medicine 88)	Mary C. Rawlinson	Shannon Lundeen		978-1-4020-4508-0
89	2006-06-27	Bormuth, Life Conduct in Modern Times (Philosophy and Medicine 89)	Matthias Bormuth			978-1-4020-4764-0
90	2007-03-08	Kincaid (Eds), Establishing Medical Reality (Philosophy and Medicine 90)	Harold Kincaid	Jennifer McKitrick		978-1-4020-5215-6
92	2007-04-07	Wright, Means, Ends and Medical Care (Philosophy and Medicine 92)	H.G. Wright			978-1-4020-5291-0
94	2007-09-24	Cherry (Eds), Pluralistic Casuistry (Philosophy and Medicine 94)	Mark J. Cherry	Ana Smith Iltis		978-1-4020-6259-9
97	2008-09-08	Lustig (Eds), Altering Nature (Philosophy and Medicine 97)	B. A. Lustig	B.A. Brody	Gerald P. McKenny	978-1-4020-6920-8
98	2008-07-21	Lustig (Eds), Altering Nature (Philosophy and Medicine 98)	B. A. Lustig	B.A. Brody	Gerald P. McKenny	978-1-4020-6922-2

(continued)

Volume_ number	Publication date	Short_title	Author editor 1	Author editor 2	Author editor 3	ISBN
99	2008-05-29	Marcum, An Introductory Philosophy of Medicine (Philosophy and Medicine 99)	James A. Marcum			978-1-4020-6796-9
100	2011-11-19	Engelhardt (Ed), Bioethics Critically Reconsidered (Philosophy and Medicine 100)	H. Tristram Engelhardt			978-94-007-2243-9
101	2008-09-25	Jotterand (Ed), Emerging Conceptual, Ethical and Policy Issues in Bionanotechnology (Philosophy and Medicine 101)	Fabrice Jotterand			978-1-4020-8648-9
102	2009-01-09	IP (Ed), The Bioethics of Regenerative Medicine (Philosophy and Medicine 102)	King-Tak IP			978-1-4020-8966-4
103	2009-10-01	Hanson, Moral Acquaintances and Moral Decisions (Philosophy and Medicine 103)	Stephen S. Hanson			978-90-481-2507-4
104	2009-10-21	Ralston (Eds), Philosophical Reflections on Disability (Philosophy and Medicine 104)	D. Christopher Ralston	Justin Ho		978-90-481-2476-3
106	2010-02-04	Pessini (Eds), Ibero-American Bioethics (Philosophy and Medicine 106)	Léo Pessini	Christian Paul de Barchifontaine	Fernando Lolas Stepke	978-1-4020-9349-4
107	2010-06-06	Roberts, Abortion and the Moral Significance of Merely Possible Persons (Philosophy and Medicine 107)	Melinda A. Roberts			978-90-481-3791-6
108	2010-06-25	DiSilvestro, Human Capacities and Moral Status (Philosophy and Medicine 108)	Russell DiSilvestro			978-90-481-8536-8
109	2010-12-15	Wiggins (Eds), Clinical Ethics and the Necessity of Stories (Philosophy and Medicine 109)	Osborne P. Wiggins	Annette C. Allen		978-90-481-9189-5
110	2010-11-11	Tollefsen (Ed), Bioethics with Liberty and Justice (Philosophy and Medicine 110)	Christopher Tollefsen			978-90-481-9790-3
113	2011-09-28	Sadegh-Zadeh, Handbook of Analytic Philosophy of Medicine (Philosophy and Medicine 113)	Kazem Sadegh-Zadeh			978-94-007-2259-0
114	2012-01-03	Marcum, The Virtuous Physician (Philosophy and Medicine 114)	James A. Marcum			978-94-007-2705-2

115	2013-01-02	Garrett (Eds), The Development of Bioethics in the United States (Philosophy and Medicine 115)	Jeremy R. Garrett	Fabrice Jotterand	D. Christopher Ralston	978-94-007-4010-5
117	2016-07-06	Sobiech, Ethos, Bioethics, and Sexual Ethics in Work and Reception of the Anatomist Niels Stensen (1638-1686) (Philosophy and Medicine 117)	Frank Sobiech			978-3-319-32911-6
118	2015-01-20	Reach, The Mental Mechanisms of Patient Adherence to Long-Term Therapies (Philosophy and Medicine 118)	Gérard Reach			978-3-319-12264-9
119	2015-04-27	Sadegh-Zadeh, Handbook of Analytic Philosophy of Medicine (Philosophy and Medicine 119), 2nd ed.	Kazem Sadegh-Zadeh			978-94-017-9578-4
120	2015-06-09	Meacham (Ed), Medicine and Society, New Perspectives in Continental Philosophy (Philosophy and Medicine 120)	Darian Meacham			978-94-017-9869-3
122	2017-03-03	Ho (Ed), Philosophical Issues in Pharmaceutics (Philosophy and Medicine 122)	Dien Ho			978-94-024-0977-2
123	2017-05-05	Stolberg, A History of Palliative Care, 1500-1970 (Philosophy and Medicine 123)	Michael Stolberg			978-3-319-54177-8
124	2016-10-19	Fanning, Normative and Pragmatic Dimensions of Genetic Counseling (Philosophy and Medicine 124)	Joseph B. Fanning			978-3-319-44928-9
125	2015-10-30	Rasmussen (Eds), At the Foundations of Bioethics and Biopolitics: Critical Essays on the Thought of H. Tristram Engelhardt, Jr. (Philosophy and Medicine 125)	Lisa M. Rasmussen	Ana Iltis	Mark J. Cherry	978-3-319-18964-2
126	2017-06-01	Quante, Personal Identity as a Principle of Biomedical Ethics (Philosophy and Medicine 126)	Michael Quante			978-3-319-56867-6
128	2018-05-07	Soniewicka (Ed), The Ethics of Reproductive Genetics (Philosophy and Medicine 128)	Marta Soniewicka			978-3-319-60683-5
129	2018-08-27	Watson (Eds), Moral Expertise (Philosophy and Medicine 129)	Jamie Carlin Watson	Laura K. Guidry-Grimes		978-3-319-92758-9

(continued)

Volume_ number	Publication date	Short_title	Author editor 1	Author editor 2	Author editor 3	ISBN
130	2019-03-19	Cataldo (Eds), Palliative Care and Catholic Health Care (Philosophy and Medicine 130)	Peter J. Cataldo	Dan O'Brien		978-3-030-05004-7
131	2019-10-08	Delimata, Articulating Intersex: A Crisis at the Intersection of Scientific Facts and Social Ideals (Philosophy and Medicine 131)	Natalie Delimata			978-3-030-21897-3
132	2023-01-03	Zima (Eds), Medical Research Ethics: Challenges in the 21st Century (Philosophy and Medicine 132)	Tomas Zima	David N. Weisstub		978-3-031-12691-8
133	2023-05-03	Fan (Ed), Incentives and Disincentives in Organ Donation (Philosophy and Medicine 133)	Ruiping Fan			978-3-031-29238-5
134	2020-06-11	Rasmussen (Ed), Human Guinea Pigs, by Kenneth Mellanby: A Reprint with Commentaries (Philosophy and Medicine 134)	Lisa M. Rasmussen			978-3-030-37696-3
135	2019-11-28	Ramm, Medical Jurisprudence and Rules of the Medical Profession (Philosophy and Medicine 135)		Rudolf Ramm		978-3-030-25244-1
136	2020-05-13	Emmerich (Eds), Contemporary European Perspectives on the Ethics of End of Life Care (Philosophy and Medicine 136)	Nathan Emmerich	Pierre Mallia	Bert Gordijn	978-3-030-40032-3
137	2022-08-28	al-Akiti (Eds), Islam and Biomedicine (Philosophy and Medicine 137)	Afifi al-Akiti	Aasim I. Padela		978-3-030-53800-2
138	2021-02-09	Cléro, Reflections on Medical Ethics (Philosophy and Medicine 138)	Jean-Pierre Cléro			978-3-030-65232-6
139	2021-08-04	Victor (Eds), Applying Nonideal Theory to Bioethics (Philosophy and Medicine 139)	Elizabeth Victor	Laura K. Guidry-Grimes		978-3-030-72502-0
140	2022-02-02	Delkeskamp-Hayes (Ed), From Physicians' Professional Ethos towards Medical Ethics and Bioethics (Philosophy and Medicine 140)	Corinna Delkeskamp-Hayes			978-3-030-78035-7

141	2022-01-19	Seidlein (Eds), Ethical Challenges for Healthcare Practices at the End of Life: Interdisciplinary Perspectives (Philosophy and Medicine 141)	Anna-Henrikje Seidlein	Sabine Salloch		978-3-030-83185-1
142	2022-04-05	McCullough, Thomas Percival's Medical Ethics and the Invention of Medical Professionalism (Philosophy and Medicine 142)	Laurence B. McCullough			978-3-030-86035-6
143	2022-07-02	Wasson (Eds), Thorny Issues in Clinical Ethics Consultation (Philosophy and Medicine 143)	Katherine Wasson	Mark Kuczewski		978-3-030-91915-3
144	2022-07-02	Schües (Eds), Stem Cell Transplantations Between Siblings as Social Phenomena (Philosophy and Medicine 144)	Christina Schües	Christoph Rehmann-Sutter	Martina Jürgensen	978-3-031-04165-5
145	2023-02-08	Curtis-Wendlandt, Chasing Tourette's: Time, Freedom, and the Missing Self (Philosophy and Medicine 145)	Lisa Curtis-Wendlandt			978-3-031-19103-9
146	2023-10-02	Anderson (Ed), Ethical Issues in Community and Patient Stakeholder–Engaged Health Research (Philosophy and Medicine 146)	Emily E. Anderson			978-3-031-40378-1
147	2023-09-21	Karhausen, The Fragility of Philosophy of Medicine (Philosophy and Medicine 147)	Lucien Karhausen			978-3-031-41632-3
148	2023-10-22	Boublil (Eds), The Vulnerability of the Human World (Philosophy and Medicine 148)	Elodie Boublil	Susi Ferrarello		978-3-031-41823-5
149		Sherlock, Medicine and Hope: A Natural Theology of Human Caretaking (Philosophy and Medicine 151)	Richard Sherlock			

GPSR Compliance
The European Union's (EU) General Product Safety Regulation (GPSR) is a set of rules that requires consumer products to be safe and our obligations to ensure this.

If you have any concerns about our products, you can contact us on

ProductSafety@springernature.com

In case Publisher is established outside the EU, the EU authorized representative is:

Springer Nature Customer Service Center GmbH
Europaplatz 3
69115 Heidelberg, Germany

www.ingramcontent.com/pod-product-compliance
Lightning Source LLC
Chambersburg PA
CBHW071947130825
31062CB00003BA/46
9783031951749